THE
GREEN
SMOOTHIES DIET

THE
GREEN
SMOOTHIES DIET

The Natural Program
for Extraordinary Health

Robyn Openshaw

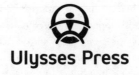

Ulysses Press

Published by: Ulysses Press
      P.O. Box 3440
      Berkeley, CA 94703
      www.ulyssespress.com

ISBN: 978-1-56975-702-4
Library of Congress Control Number: 2008911758

Printed in Canada by Marquis Book Printing

20 19 18 17 16 15 14 13 12 11

Acquisitions Editor: Nicholas Denton-Brown
Managing Editor: Claire Chun
Editors: Jennifer Privateer, Lily Chou
Editorial and production staff: Lauren Harrison, Judith Metzener,
    Elyce Petker
Cover design: what!design @ whatweb.com
Cover photos: © istockphoto.com

Distributed by Publishers Group West

NOTE TO READERS: This book has been written and published strictly for informational and educational purposes only. It is not intended to serve as medical advice or to be any form of medical treatment. You should always consult your physician before altering or changing any aspect of your medical treatment and/or undertaking a diet regimen, including the guidelines as described in this book. Do not stop or change any prescription medications without the guidance and advice of your physician. Any use of the information in this book is made on the reader's good judgment after consulting with his or her physician and is the reader's sole responsibility. This book is not intended to diagnose or treat any medical condition and is not a substitute for a physician.

    This book is independently authored and published and no sponsorship or endorsement of this book by, and no affiliation with, any trademarked brands or other products mentioned within is claimed or suggested. All trademarks that appear in ingredient lists and elsewhere in this book belong to their respective owners and are used here for informational purposes only. The authors and publishers encourage readers to patronize the quality brands mentioned and pictured in this book.

To Kincade, Emma, Mary Elizabeth, and Tennyson.
Thank you for your patience with all the "first tries."
I love and appreciate you and am blessed to be your mom
beyond my vocabulary's limited ability to express.

Contents

Introduction

In 2008, Pixar Animation Studios released a movie called
WALL-E that enthralled my four children, ages eight to fifteen.
In the movie, Earth has been abandoned by all humans
because they've so decimated their habitat with overconsumption that it's no longer habitable.

Garbage and toxic waste are everywhere. A robot named
WALL-E is the only life on the planet, and his task is to con-
solidate garbage. Meanwhile, a giant spaceship hovering over
Earth houses the remaining humans. They are so spoiled with
electronic entertainment and fast food that they no longer
work, read, or play. They float around on hover chairs, too
obese to walk, and if they fall out of the hover chairs, they
shout helplessly until robots lever them back into their chairs
and fetch them another milkshake.

The humans send a probe to Earth to try to discover any
green life remaining. The probe is appropriately named
"EVE," the archetypal "mother of all living." The surviving
humans find hope for being saved, and are able to return to
Earth, only when EVE finds a tiny green plant. Reminiscent of
the biblical story of Noah, like the dove returning with an

olive branch to signal the end of the flood, EVE returns to the ship with her tiny plant, to much rejoicing. (The crowd standing around the small plant triumphantly says, "We'll plant vegetable plants! And pizza plants!")

The fate of the entire world hangs on whether a little green plant may have survived. Granted, this is fiction, but what is the moral of the story?

In 2009, we now refer to anything that preserves our planet and slows our dreadful overconsumption habits as "green."

And yet, despite our progress as environmentalists, most American children still eat no greens, ever. Research repeatedly yields the fact that vegetable consumption by our children is an abysmal one serving per day or less, and most of the vegetables that are, in fact, eaten by our children are potatoes in the form of French fries or potato chips.

How far off, really, are we from the fate depicted in fiction such as *WALL-E*? We live in a historic age where potatoes coated in chemicals and fried in toxic trans fats qualify as the highest nutrition most children eat in a day. Unless you count the "vegetable" that is the corn-syrup-heavy ketchup that those French fries are dipped in.

Mothers know instinctively, or perhaps from long tradition, to tell their children, "Don't forget to eat your greens!" Or perhaps that's just a cliché, and today's generation of young mothers are the first *not* to say that. After all, how can they, if the mothers themselves are eating none, besides the occasional wilted piece of iceberg lettuce in a burger?

Why does this all matter? This book is my effort to document why "going green," becoming environmentally conscious, and safeguarding our health must include careful examination of the quantity of green food that we eat. We'll discuss how the key to our health does, in fact, lie in the little green plant. It lies in our ability to eat plentifully of the little green plants nature provided, taking their chlorophyll and their life force in the packages of enzymes, as well as their vitamins, minerals, and fiber.

We'll discover a way to continue to live in this fast-paced, stressful world, but easily and with little time required, getting back to our roots of eating a wide variety of greens and other plants. In so doing, we'll reduce our carbon footprint, abuse animals less, consume fewer resources, contribute to the success of local growers, as well as dramatically increase our own health and abundant living.

My interest in writing this book began in my own, very personal experience, which I share with you next. I saw my family's lives change with the habit I teach here. I have felt compelled—called, really—to share the experience I've had. I've already done so with GreenSmoothieGirl.com, and have seen thousands lose weight, regain their energy, begin digesting their food fully for the first time in their adult lives, eliminate disease, and achieve new, transcendent states of emotional and mental peace. All from a simple little habit that takes ten minutes a day.

2

My Story

To understand how I came to be a whole-foods enthusiast and educator, I really have to go back two generations.

I was blessed to be raised by people who understood the value of a natural lifestyle. My grandmother did, even while surrounded by the early love affair Americans had with pills prescribed by medical doctors and a diet of processed food and abundant animal products. The 1950s occurred long before the information age. Truly, no one had any idea that drinking Cokes and milkshakes in the local diner, eating TV dinners at home, and scarfing down lots of what Ray Kroc served up at the Golden Arches was anything but American and patriotic. Everyone did it. My own grandparents and parents resisted pop culture's obsession with addictive bad foods to an impressive extent, but, like everyone else, they somewhat indulged in the pastimes and habits of the day.

My mother's parents owned a produce dealership servicing the southern states of Arizona, New Mexico, and Texas. They had large warehouses and trucks full of fruits and vegetables 365 days a year. This made for an interesting environment that has had positive effects for a couple of generations, tapering off only now—that is, they were constantly trying to use up produce from the warehouses. Family legend has it that as my six uncles (and my dad, even though he was not yet married to my mom) loaded trucks in the warehouses during the summer, they'd purposefully drop watermelons on the asphalt because the rule was that you could eat the inventory only if it became unfit to ship.

Imagine rooms full of lettuce, spinach, pears, grapes, potatoes, jicama, carrots, grapefruit, and so much more available year-round. This is the world my parents and grandparents grew up in. They didn't really know it at the time, but my six uncles and my mom—and my six great-uncles and my grandfather—had access to the ultimate disease-minimizing diet. They were constantly trying to eat produce before it went bad. They rarely ate meat; for them, meat and dairy products were expensive, whereas produce was virtually free.

Fast forward to the next generation. My mother raised a large family of eight children (including six sons!) on an almost-exclusively plant-based diet. Although she was ahead of her time, she did this not because she understood the health implications, but rather because, unlike the rest of America, she'd never developed a love affair with animal flesh. She didn't even know how to cook a steak, an event that never happened once as I was growing up. On a rare occasion, she'd serve something with hamburger or chicken in it.

Mostly, we ate green salads and fruit for dinner, with potatoes or legumes (beans) of some kind. As a teenager, I learned to make six loaves of homemade whole-wheat bread every week, with wheat and soybeans I ground myself in our big Magic Mill grinder that sounded like a jet engine in the garage. For school lunch, while my peers ate greasy pizza, we had the same thing every day: a peanut butter sandwich with that dense whole-grain bread, an apple, and a carrot. For breakfast, we ate homemade oatmeal or Cream of Wheat, a ration of really awful-tasting unsweetened grapefruit juice from the military commissary, and a big handful of vitamins.

Looking back, I realize that my mother did a brilliant job feeding a family of ten on an Air Force officer's single income. She didn't really care that all my friends had Twinkies and Doritos accompanying their bologna-on-white-bread sandwiches every day. I deeply resented that I didn't have a thermos full of Kool-Aid like my friends did. But my mother, currently in her late 60s, very spry and running around Europe doing community service, stayed the course. I'll be eternally grateful for that example, and for her mother's example as well.

Of course, much less was known about health at that time than is known now. My mother and her parents did, in fact, live in that dearth of information, before the toll on the public health of 21st-century living began to catch up with us all and become obvious. In the 1950s, we were just beginning to see a rise in heart disease, cancer, diabetes, and other diseases. A few decades later, public health officials would be ringing the alarm bell. But, at the time, Americans were, by and large, oblivious. My mom didn't make dessert often. When she did, it was chocolate chip cookies with whole-wheat flour and the sugar and butter cut in half. But she did serve Jell-O for every fancy meal. She did become addicted to Dr. Pepper as a teenager and young adult.

My maternal grandmother was diagnosed with a very deadly melanoma when she was only 53 years old. My grandmother was a force of nature. She was never one to worry about what everyone else was doing. She consulted with medical doctors and was told that her cancer was 95 percent fatal. Still, in a gutsy move I'm to this day in awe of, she said "no thanks" to the prescribed chemotherapy and radiation. This was around 1980, long before anyone in the mainstream had heard of the raw-food diet, before anyone, really, had begun to question modern medicine's cancer protocols. Even then, with a support system of exactly no one, she knew she didn't want to cut, burn, and poison herself to remove the deadly growth.

Instead, she undertook her own design of natural protocols. She studied on her own and consulted with practitioners outside the medical profession. She followed what logic, observation, and intuition told her to do, even while everyone around her, including most of her own children, felt she was crazy.

Specifically, she went to Southern California to get help at Optimum Health Institute, founded by the late, great nutrition pioneer Ann Wigmore (Wigmore promoted wheatgrass juice and a raw, plant-based diet decades before large-scale studies underpinned what she was teaching). Grandmother also went to Mexico to obtain laetrile, a compound in apricot pits rich in B12 that was banned in the U.S. Then she began eating a raw, plant-food diet. She juiced daily, and drank so many carrots that her skin turned orange from the beta-carotene.

As our large family watched, astonished, she healed herself of cancer. The theory behind the raw-food movement, in its most incipient stage at that time, is that cancer cannot live in the presence of oxygen. As you fully oxygenate the blood and, subsequently, the tissues and cells, you starve cancer out. I've watched a number of friends do this successfully in the ensuing years.

But my grandmother was far ahead of her time, and she undertook this regimen against great opposition. She went on to travel the world, greet her 49 grandchildren and some of her great grandchildren as they came into the world, and complete five international service missions for 25 more years. Much later in life, having relaxed her nutritional standards very significantly, different forms of cancer came back and took both her and my grandfather in their late 70s. When my grandfather's cancer was diagnosed at age 75, his medical doctor said that it had been growing so slowly for 30 years only because of his excellent diet. He was on that diet with my grandmother as she healed herself many years before, and it maintained their good health for many years afterward.

That my grandmother's anti-cancer diet also gave my grandfather many years of life is an example of how although we may be targeting a specific health issue with nutrition, along the way we realize that nutrition has benefits we could have never even dreamed up. It's just part of what is so exciting about returning to a diet of eating low on the food chain.

My grandmother's cancer story happened while I was in high school, at the same time that another dramatic event unfolded in my family. My uncle (the middle of my mother's six brothers) was diagnosed at 32 years of age with a very treatable, stage 1 Hodgkin's disease. Hodgkin's is a cancer of the lymphatic system. My uncle was told by his oncologist, as my grandmother (who was with him) reported, "I guarantee that if you follow this protocol [of chemotherapy and radiation treatment], you will recover."

Eighteen months later, physically devastated, bedridden, debilitated, and weighing much less than 100 pounds, my uncle died a very awful death from the side effects of the treatment. He left behind his wonderful wife, three small children, and a stunned and devastated extended family.

This is a delicate issue that deeply divided my mother's family. To this day, some believe that my grandparents died needlessly in their late 70s because they chose to forego standard medical care. My grandparents had decided they would rather let cancer take them than submit to the cutting-and-burning methodologies. Others believe that my uncle's death was God's will. I don't wish to refute any of those beliefs, as I'm not the arbiter of truth, and all those opinions and feelings in my extended family are deeply held and valid.

The point is that, at a very young age, I became aware of the limitations of medical practice. I became a believer that diet is powerful medicine.

That is where my story begins. At the time, I was less than supportive of my mother's culinary habits. I was mortified when she'd invite people who'd stopped by to come in for dinner. "Dinner" was simply a bowl of boiled new potatoes with sour cream, a bowl of sliced cantaloupe, and a big romaine salad. After I got married, at the age of 21, to a 6'4" college football offensive lineman, my new husband was horrified by the menu. He thought he'd starve to death eating like that.

He'd come from a meat-and-potatoes family: animal protein was served at virtually every meal, and processed foods like white flour and sugar were embraced. His family bought nacho cheese sauce in number-ten cans and served pies cut in fourths as standard serving sizes. He didn't feel the meals I cooked were truly meals without the meat.

However, he couldn't help but be impressed when, as he began eating my cooking, his high blood pressure immediately dropped to ideal levels and he lost 40 pounds. His being healthy and fit was especially striking, not only in his family, who struggles with heart disease, cancer, gout, arthritis, being overweight, and other issues, but also in football's lineman culture, where the vast majority of his peers became very overweight after college and stayed that way. We're in our early 40s and very recently have lost a couple of his former football buddies to preventable, lifestyle-related diseases.

But, like my mother, I didn't know how to cook meat and hadn't been conditioned to expect a slab of it on my plate at dinner. In fact, early in my marriage, I went to a three-day campout with my husband's family. The campfire menus included meat (much of it processed) three times a day. I was worried about offending, so I ate what I was served.

I can count on one hand the times I've thrown up in my life. But, after one day of that, my body sent me a message, and I threw up after my third meat-based meal. I decided to eat only whatever plant foods I could find for the rest of the campout. My nutrition views were not particularly welcomed, nor had I developed the skills at age 21 to really convert anyone, so I kept my opinions to myself for the remainder of our 20-year marriage.

While I'd been shown a path that was much better than the standard American diet, I did veer way off course. In my 20s, I embraced a fairly typical American diet. I gained 15 pounds the first year of my desk job out of college. When I got pregnant at 26, I indulged in my very own "Supersize Me" experiment. We sat in a La-Z Boy, watching TV every night and eating Ben & Jerry's Cookie Dough ice cream. I ate a burger and fries special for 99 cents every day at lunch in the company cafeteria. Anything green sounded revolting, especially in the queasy first trimester, so I didn't bother.

Once I had an overwhelming Diet Coke craving and went to the 7-11 and got a Big Gulp. The baby inside me shook for hours afterward. (I did vow never to do that again.) My blood pressure, always about 95/55, rose to 120/80. I gained 65 pounds. My ankles swelled up with edema to the point where, as a trick at parties, I'd push my finger in and watch how the depression in my ankles stayed there for 30 seconds. I developed hemorrhoids and terrible blood sugar problems. I once saw a former boyfriend as I was walking through the mall and said hello, but my face was so fat he just gave me a strange look and kept walking. He had no idea who I was. (And I was instantly glad, after realizing that I didn't want to be recognized anyway.) Sometimes I show these photos when I teach a nutrition class.

I hated what had happened to my formerly athletic and lean body. I lost the weight within six months of having my first baby, and had healthier pregnancies thereafter. When my little boy Kincade was seven months old, I made my first very major mistake as a parent. I weaned him from nursing to baby formula. He immediately began to be constantly ill, with colds, chest congestion, and a green, snotty nose. He'd be up all night unable to breathe, coughing constantly. The illness would subside but come back with a vengeance. He was sick off and on, constantly. We'd pump him full of cough medicine and sit up all night rocking him. Eventually, at 12 months, according to doctor recommendations, we moved from cow's-milk formula, to plain old cow's milk.

We were in and out of the pediatrician's office constantly. When Kincade was a little over a year old, the pediatrician told me that based on how often he came to the office with wheezing problems, he had asthma. I was devastated. I had mental images of a pale, sickly kid sitting on the sidelines at a soccer game sucking on an inhaler.

The first time I'd been to the pediatrician and been given the diagnosis, I'd asked, "What is asthma?" The doctor said, very slowly, as if I were stupid, "It's a luuuuung diseeeease." I smiled and said I understood that. "But what is it, exactly?" He pulled a brochure from a drug company from a plastic wall dispenser and handed it to me. That was my education.

I was very unsatisfied with both that "help" my insurance company readily paid for, as well as the five courses of steroids that were prescribed to my son in that first year after he began getting sick. When the fifth round was diagnosed, the pediatrician mentioned to me, offhandedly, "By the way, we know from research that children who have at least five rounds of steroids a year are guaranteed to have stunted growth." Shocked, I asked about that in more detail, and he said, "Well, we can't do studies on it, really. That would be unethical, to recruit human subjects when we know that the result will be stunted growth." I left the office that day not only frustrated and confused, but also upset that even though "research" on massive steroid use is "unethical," it was somehow not unethical to keep feeding them to my son.

That was, incidentally, the last prescription I would ever fill for my son. He would never again be administered antibiotics or steroids, and the bronchodilator drugs in the nebulizer machine we'd used so extensively in the middle of the night were soon to be history.

As frustrated as I was that day, it was also an epiphany. I realized in that moment, with great clarity, how unacceptably limited modern medicine's ability to help my son was. This caused a breaking point in this sick relationship I'd developed, where my son would be turning blue, and I'd call the on-call doctor or nurse and beg for help. I became aware of the narrow range of options that I'd get, no matter how sick my son might become. He'd be given pills and gaseous drugs—but nothing, absolutely nothing, besides newer drugs. I realized, with a shock, that even when his oxygen dropped and he was rushed to an emergency room and turned blue—the doctor had no magic bullet. Just more of the exact same drugs prescribed all along.

Realizing this limitation forced me to begin taking true responsibility for little Kincade's health. At first, this was terribly frightening. I had been abdicating that responsibility to someone else. I had a false sense of security because that person wore a white coat, had a bit more formal education than I did, and was graced with the built-in clout of having a waiting room full of other sick kids and desperate parents.

I have come to learn that this is a first step for many, if not all, of us when we face a health crisis. That is, we exhaust medicine's options and see it from that inside position of knowing exactly what is available. At that point, there is no more mystique, no remaining glamour. As in *The Wizard of Oz*, the wizard behind the screen is exposed as a fraud. Or, worse, as in The Emperor's New Clothes, we become aware that the emperor is not, in fact, clothed in beautiful, stylish garments, but is, rather, just plain naked. We realize that we cannot look to these gods of popular culture to save us.

And then the panic sets in. This doctor was, after all, the man I placed all my faith in, the person who was supposed to help my son when he was sick, the guy with all the education and answers.

For those of you facing a health crisis, take heart. This initial fear gave way, over the course of a long learning curve I hope to address in this book, to a sense of empowerment. With all my writing and teaching, I attempt to make that learning curve shorter for anyone wishing to learn.

Because the good news is: I now know how to recognize a healing crisis. I know which foods are truly nutritious and which aren't. (This is information that the vast majority of Americans do not have. It's not just that they lack self-discipline or make poor choices—they truly don't know because of the false and downright injurious education they have received.) I know how to heal and build my own body and my children's with nutrition. I know how to cleanse the organs of elimination whenever necessary. Most importantly, I know how to avoid the need for all that, massively reducing our risk of not only degenerative diseases like cancer and heart disease, but also of simple colds and flu, by just eating simply, low on the food chain, every day.

I don't feel afraid now of cancer and heart disease, or of a long winter of coughing and falling ill. These things simply don't happen in my home anymore. They're a distant memory.

I was able not only to obtain the learning and knowledge that would powerfully help and even heal my son, but also to be armed with tools that would change my family's health forever. I was blessed with three more children, all with the same inherent genetic weakness and propensity toward asthma. Now I know that an autoimmune disease is evidence of a few generations of genetic deterioration leading to problems that can be helped with strong nutrition. In the past few generations, by eating lots of processed foods and animal protein, we've actually altered the DNA that we're passing on to the physically weakest generation, possibly in the history of the world.

It was certainly a sea change to go into my pantry and dump all the Tupperware labeled flour, sugar, cornmeal, spaghetti—and relabel those same containers with things I'd never heard of before: quinoa, spelt, Kamut, oat groats. And also to fill up the fridge with produce and rice or almond milk instead of cow's milk.

Here are some of the quantifiable gains I've seen in my own health as a result of changing our diet, the same I teach you to do in this book:

- My children's asthma more or less disappeared; we never again needed a steroid prescription or an emergency room or emergency doctor visit.
- I lost pounds I'd been carrying for several years and achieved my ideal weight, easily and without dieting or deprivation.
- I regained energy I'd lost in my 20s and have more energy at 42 than I had at 22.
- My really scary migraines (right arm going numb, unable to see or talk for several hours) stopped.
- I needed two hours less sleep at night and no longer had chronic insomnia.
- I didn't crash into coma-like 90-minute naps in the afternoon anymore.
- I bounced out of bed in the morning instead of needing 20 minutes to drag myself out.
- Panic attacks and anxiety I'd had since childhood disappeared (and return only if I eat sugar) and my mood is more sustained, positive, and calm.
- Our digestive problems are gone: all of us are totally regular (no one has been constipated in 15 years), no hard or foul-smelling stools, eliminations are complete.

- Nobody gets sick anymore, besides an occasional mild cold (no strep, bacterial infection, or flu in ten years).
- All four kids grew strong and tall and dominate in competitive athletics.
- Menstrual irregularity disappeared, PMS symptoms dramatically lessened (I didn't get so cranky, didn't have cramps, didn't break out).
- I loved people more naturally and purely, and I took my frustrations with people in stride, even when their behaviors were negative—instead of wanting them to just leave me alone! My siblings and parents commented on the dramatic change in my personality.
- My nails lost their white spots, grew quickly, and became strong and flexible.
- My cravings for bad foods lessened (gone eventually, as long as I don't eat sugar and refined salt).
- People in the family who had warts lost them (they just went away).
- Nearly all of us had eczema, and it went away for everyone. Dry skin in the winter went away when I added coconut oil to our diet.
- Two of us had hay fever, which dramatically decreased, no longer requiring drugs.
- I used to be a terrible runner and hated it; now I look forward to running 15 to 20 miles per week and sometimes run races.
- I have aged much more slowly than my peers.
- Doctors have told me I have cardiac markers seen only in triathletes, including a resting heart rate in the 50s, very low blood pressure, and total cholesterol below 100!

- I used to wear glasses in college and, without corrective techniques or surgery, now have 20-15 vision (better than perfect) simply from dietary changes.

I've been blessed with massively improved health and a disappearance of "symptoms" for my son and the rest of the family. But even greater consequences have resulted from the path I started down in 1994. I've found a new mission in life: to help others achieve vibrant health. What started as a simple quest to help my little boy with asthma has had far-reaching consequences, I hope, for good.

I've felt called and compelled to share what I've learned, and I've been emboldened in teaching others as I've witnessed thousands who have attended my classes, followed my program *12 Steps to Whole Foods*, watched my YouTube videos, and read my blogs achieve dramatically improved health. Even more exciting to me is the quantum leap that this knowledge base takes when those following my 12-step program on Green SmoothieGirl.com and following the principles in this book inspire and teach others. So many of my readers tell me of similar stories in their own lives. As their health changes for the better, they lose weight and begin accomplishing goals long on the back burner. Others notice and ask how to do it, too.

The old Zen saying is that when a student is ready, a teacher appears. And so it happens with nutrition. Those suffering take note of the person who is experiencing vibrant health and ask her how she does it.

That is my hope for you—you've made the wise step to read a book about how to massively change your diet and lifestyle for the better, in the easiest, most high-impact way possible. My hope is that not only will you experience exciting reversal-of-aging results, you'll subsequently be a cheerleader and teacher of others. So many in this world are suffering. And that suffering is so unnecessary.

But start with you. You can't strap an oxygen mask on your neighbor, on the airplane, unless you have yours on first. We've been losing altitude, nutritionally, as a culture for a long time. It's time to right the course.

3

What I Did That Saved My Family's Health

I've written of the epiphany I had in a pediatrician's office, wherein I realized that I, not the doctor, would have to address my family's health issues. I could sit back and hope that doctors would solve our health problems, but that would be living inside a lie. The doctors were never going to solve my children's problems. On that epiphanic day, I saw that very clearly.

Watching others pursue the medical route for many years now, my initial impression has been confirmed over and over. I feel blessed now that I didn't learn this after 10, 20, or 30 years of placing ongoing, excessive faith in doctors, as I've seen many people do, who end up highly disillusioned in the end and, sometimes, severely damaged by those medical treatments.

Besides learning about a handful of herbs and natural remedies for ear infections and viral and bacterial infections, I really didn't do much besides learn extensively about nutrition and apply those principles. Sorting through all the bogus food theories out there was the first challenge. The biggest stumbling block for people currently trying to learn about how to feed themselves appropriately is the mountain of pop-culture noise in the form of the *high-protein fad*. This insidious and dangerous body of dubious advice has caused millions of people to miss the true, real, only path to durable muscle mass, weight control, disease risk minimization, energy, and wellness. And it is, indeed, a fad. It'll go away as surely as it came along. The Atkins Diet is already fading into oblivion, thankfully, even if a toxic obsession with animal protein has remained in our culture as a sick vestige of that fad.

Seeing clearly through all the information clutter allows you to dismiss these diets that disallow even whole-food carbohydrates (like whole grains) and push lots of chicken, fish, and other animal proteins. Not only is this an unnatural diet that causes us to eat far too high on the food chain, straining the Earth's ability to deliver, but it's also unacceptably disease causing.

The Oxford-Cornell China Project is the biggest nutrition study in history, called the "grand prix of epidemiology" by the *New York Times*. The study, by two of the greatest research institutions in the world, was funded for nearly 30 years, studying 6,500 people and yielding hundreds of statistically significant findings. The main discovery is that high animal-protein diets (dairy and meat) lead to high rates of cancer, heart disease, and autoimmune disorders.

Funding was obtained for this massive research project after startling findings with animals. The lead researcher, Colin Campbell, Ph.D., is one of America's most preeminent nutrition authorities. He grew up on a cattle ranch and believed originally that low-protein diets were poor diets. Early in his career, he went to the Philippines to study children with liver cancer, anticipating that poor children without access to animal protein would be overrepresented in the cancer group. In fact, the opposite was the case: The relatively affluent children with access to meat and dairy were the ones getting cancer in alarming numbers.

Campbell moved on to studies with mice and rats. The mice fed a 5-percent-casein (milk protein) diet lived past their prime, running in their wheels, lean and vigorous and free of tumors. The rodents fed a 20-percent-animal-protein diet died early after becoming overweight and sluggish, refusing to run in the hamster wheels, and growing cancerous tumors. Both groups were fed the cancer-initiating toxic compound aflatoxin, but only the animal-protein-fed animals actually grew tumors!

Possibly even more fascinating and compelling is that mid-study, the researchers switched the diets. The overweight, tumor-ridden mice were switched to a 5-percent-animal-protein diet. Their tumors shrunk, they outlived the cancerous mice from the previous study group, and became lean and healthy again.

On the other hand, the lean mice formerly fed a mostly plant-based diet (5 percent animal protein) were switched to a 20-percent-protein diet. They gained weight, grew tumors, and died. This study was repeated by other, unrelated researchers in other places around the globe, thus documenting the highest standards in research, reliability, and validity. That is, the studies were repeated with consistent results, and they were, in fact, measuring what they set out to measure, as variable control was simple to obtain.

Dr. Joel Fuhrman, M.D., author of *Eat to Live* and other books, has stated that we now have more evidence that meat and dairy cause disease than we have evidence that smoking causes lung cancer! This may be hard for some to believe, until one begins to study the mountain of empirical evidence for which the Oxford-Cornell Project simply put the final nail in the coffin. The intent of this book is not to cover that deluge of data, but a few of my favorite sources can help anyone suffering from cognitive dissonance over this claim that animal protein diets make us ill.

Consider some of these preeminent, qualified voices from just this decade who review in detail why raw plant food, especially green plant food, rather than animal flesh, is the answer to our health problems:

- T. Colin Campbell, Ph.D., *The China Study* (2004)
- Joel Fuhrman, M.D., *Eat to Live* (2003) and *Disease-Proof Your Child* (2006)
- John Robbins, *The Food Revolution* (2001)
- Robert O. Young, Ph.D., *Sick and Tired* (2001)
- Gabriel Cousens, M.D., *Rainbow Green Live-Food Cuisine* (2003)
- Caldwell Esselstyn, M.D.
- John McDougall, M.D.
- Neal Barnard, M.D.

For many people, letting go of the idea that we must have quantities of animal protein for health is like switching religions. These beliefs have been around so pervasively during our generation that the belief we need our "protein" runs bone-deep.

Still, I've seen many die-hard, lifelong meat eaters change their diets dramatically toward a mostly raw, plant-based diet and begin to look like literally different people. They become healthier, leaner, more physically and spiritually beautiful people with clearer skin and a vibrance that people notice. The raw, plant-based diet movement has so many converts, primarily because of the undeniable results you witness in the gorgeous people who eat mostly raw and alkaline foods for many years. This includes actress Demi Moore, bestselling author and life coach Tony Robbins, supermodel Carol Alt, and my friend, the breast cancer survivor Shelley Abegg, who is 50 years old but looks 30. They don't all eat identical diets (Carol Alt eats raw animal products, for instance, in addition to mostly plants, and Tony Robbins focuses on eating alkaline foods). However, regardless of these differences, what they all have in common is they all eat enzyme-rich, power-packed raw greens, vegetables, and fruits daily.

So let's get to what you really want to know: In 1994 I began eating a primarily plant-based diet. To this day, I eat the foods in the pyramid below. They're given in this order because they are, from top to bottom, the highest-quantity ingredient in the diet to the lowest quantity. Eating in this way focuses on foods that are the most nutrient dense—that is, the highest

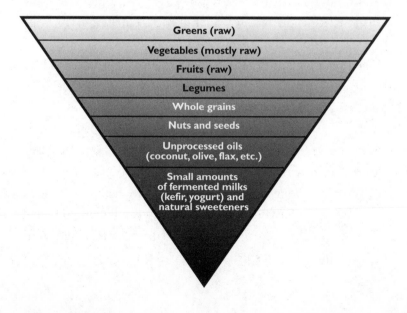

Greens (raw)

Vegetables (mostly raw)

Fruits (raw)

Legumes

Whole grains

Nuts and seeds

Unprocessed oils
(coconut, olive, flax, etc.)

Small amounts
of fermented milks
(kefir, yogurt) and
natural sweeteners

micronutrients (vitamins and minerals) for the lowest calories, plus small amounts of good fats.

This may seem like a boring or restrictive diet. It comprises, however, hundreds of foods entailing thousands of possibilities for recipes, including main dishes, salads, dressings, sauces, salsas, soups, crackers, snacks, smoothies, and desserts. In the past ten years, a very exciting information age has begun in nutrition: You have thousands of recipes available from gourmet cooks—anything from the simple to the complex—utilizing what is now known about nutrition.

By learning this information, you unlock the secrets to health with keys that were completely unavailable to your parents and grandparents unless they were lucky enough to stumble upon seriously counterculture, lone pioneer voices such as Ann Wigmore or Bernard Jensen. Your parents and grandparents blindly accepted the products of Coca-Cola and Betty Crocker and Swanson without having any idea what the ramifications were to their health.

You and I are blessed to live in that moment in time unparalleled in history in which massive nutritional information, based on real science, has converged with the means to obtain fresh produce and other whole foods. For thousands of years, many people of the Earth, while they had no access to processed foods, also had little access to fresh, whole foods during the winter. We should, because of our fortuitous circumstances, be the healthiest people in the history of the world. The only thing standing in our way is our choices.

What will your choices be? That you're reading this book is a good sign that you're on your way to capitalizing on what is known in the information age about how to reach your physical, mental, and spiritual potential through lifestyle.

4

Why Green Foods?

Green foods are very likely the most nutritionally precise foods to meet the needs of human beings. Let's look at the ways they are the perfect food to nourish every cell, prevent risk, and keep us lean and energetic.

Protein

Let's begin with protein, since people in the Western world are rather preoccupied with this topic (needlessly, I should add, since nature provides foods that have absolutely perfect protein/carb/fat proportions). Certainly protein (along with carbohydrates and fats) is needed in our diet and is, indeed, very important to build muscle mass and maintain the health of tissues throughout the body.

When I ask my classes whether they think beef or spinach is higher in protein, calorie for calorie, they can see a trick question coming, but they generally go with what they know—that red meat, of course, is the gold standard in protein. But it isn't true. Red meat is a "perfect" protein, which doesn't mean what the public assumes it means, that it's somehow a *better* protein than, for instance, what is found abundantly in greens and vegetables. A perfect protein is simply one that matches human flesh very closely. The kind found in greens, like spinach, consists of much more loosely arranged amino acids, which the body has to work a bit harder to assemble.

People are consistently shocked to learn that, for instance, broccoli and spinach are more than 40 percent protein. But protein content is only one of the ways that greens are easily the most perfect, nourishing, disease-preventing foods anywhere on Planet Earth.

I have programmed my green smoothie ingredients into calorie- and nutrition-calculators, and they average about 9 to 10 percent protein, which is ideal. The 20 percent protein target of Barry Sears (the Zone Diet) and others is counter to what is natural, and it's the amount of protein in the standard American diet. It's also the amount of protein, exactly, in the China Study groups of rats, mice, and people who were at highest risk for disease. An 80/10/10 ratio of carbs/protein/fats is much more ideal and more in keeping with what is found in nature and good for the use of humans.

If you're looking to increase protein in your plant foods for a specific health reason, consider that spinach is highest, at 42 percent protein, and use it liberally in your green smoothies (while also getting a variety of greens). Try to make your smoothies as low in fruit as possible for your own taste, and consider making the no-fruit smoothie at the beginning of the recipe chapter at the end of this book.

You can certainly add protein powder, though most whey- and soy-based protein powders are fractionated, heat-treated, and not good for you. Many studies in the past decade show that soy is not the health food we thought it was for many years. Soy in its whole and fermented forms, used in moderation, are likely entirely appropriate. The problem is that we're being bombarded with far too much soy in the form of processed isolates (parts of the grain separated from the whole food). Soy lecithin, soy proteins, and many other derivatives are in thousands of grocery store offerings. Please avoid soy protein powders. And we've already discussed how the casein in whey is the protein base used in Campbell's animal studies in *The China Study* that, in typical American proportions, lead to cancer, heart disease, and many other diseases.

The best protein powder, for nutrition as well as taste, is SunWarrior's fermented brown-rice protein powder, which can be obtained online. My second choice would be hemp protein powder, available at health food stores, though it's lower in protein and a bit grittier. I often eat a handful of sprouted, dehydrated almonds with my green smoothie for a very satisfying lunch with plenty of protein.

I don't think anyone knows exactly what seven-time Tour de France winner Lance Armstrong's diet is. But if you read his story written by his nutrition coach, you know a couple of things.

First, he eats 70 percent carbs, 15 percent protein, and 15 percent fat. You'd have a very hard time attaining that without a heavily plant-based diet. I wonder if that has also been a factor in Mr. Armstrong's cancer not returning. Second, the team keeps turbo blenders on the bus for making smoothies after each race. Green smoothies, maybe?

In addition to the plant-based diet of Tony Gonzalez (the Kansas City Chiefs' tight end), Salim Stoudamire (Atlanta Hawks' guard) and Ultimate Fighting champion Mac Danzi, these athletes were vegetarians:

- Bill Pearl, who had the longest and most successful career in bodybuilding;
- Martina Navratilova, who dominated women's tennis for 20 years and played for 30;
- Edwin Moses, who won 122 races over the course of ten years;
- Carl Lewis, who won nine gold medals in four Olympiads;
- Hank Aaron, who holds the home-run record in baseball.

One thing that these athletes have in common is endurance in their sports, much longer than the average pro. This is just more evidence that plant food (especially raw) is the fountain of youth, providing all known nutritional compounds to slow aging and energy maintenance for life.

Chlorophyll and blood-building properties

One of the reasons greens are powerhouse foods is the plant energy derived from chlorophyll, which is the plant equivalent of hemoglobin in the human red blood cell. Chlorophyll neutralizes internal body odors and bad breath, and it mops up free radicals that cause cancer and all degenerative disease.

Calcium

Everyone knows that calcium (combined with vitamin D obtained by spending a moderate amount of time in the sun) builds strong bones. Many people think that dairy products are their best sources of calcium. In fact, while dairy is high in calcium, it's not particularly bioavailable to human beings. The foods highest in calcium highly useable by people are, of course, greens. Highest are collards, parsley, watercress, dandelion greens, beet greens, and kale.

Unparalleled nutritional profile

Greens are a powerhouse of enzymes, vitamins, and minerals. They are, ounce for ounce, the most nutritionally dense foods on the planet because they're the lowest in calories and highest in micronutrients. Scientists have recently discovered a number of nutritional classes of micronutrient compounds, but we still don't know how they all work together to protect against cancer and disease. What we do know is that greens, unlike synthetic vitamins, contain those compounds that synergistically reduce our risk of myriad health problems.

Most leafy greens are extremely high in antioxidant vitamins A, C, and E that bind with and neutralize free radicals. They're a source of folic acid that helps prevent birth defects in babies, as well as magnesium, which is an easy nutrient to become deficient in. Their dark colors show that they're high in phytochemicals, including over 500 carotenoid antioxidants, flavonoids, and indoles working synergistically to give the eater of greens abundant health. No supplement can provide the perfect balance of nutrition that raw green food contains naturally.

Fiber

Millions of Americans depend on chemical derivative fiber supplements to compensate for their low-fiber diet. (Chemical drinks like Metamucil are not the same as natural plant fiber and can irritate and overstimulate your body's digestive system.) This is a tragedy with epic consequences, not least of which is skyrocketing colon cancer deaths. The colon will be healthy if we provide it, all day long, with lots of insoluble plant fiber. That bulk drags the length of our gastrointestinal tract, much like a broom, keeping its tissues clean and pink and healthy.

Fiber famously prevents all types of cancers and digestive problems, but it also reduces cholesterol and heart disease, and controls blood sugar by slowing sugar uptake in the bloodstream. It prevents gallstones, decreases diabetes risk, binds excess estrogen, and assists in weight loss by creating a sense of fullness and less desire to overeat.

You don't find many foods higher in fiber than greens. The insoluble fiber functions like a sponge in the gut, and can expand, soak up, and remove several times its own weight in toxic materials. Its importance cannot be overstated because it's the only way we have to move dead cells and many other wastes through the body in minimal time, avoiding the decomposing and diseased cells that result when food sits, undigested, in various parts of our digestive and elimination systems.

A quart or more of green smoothie daily is a phenomenal way to dramatically increase fiber in the diet. A quart should provide 12–15 grams of fiber to your diet. The average American gets only 11 grams of fiber daily, so if you're coming from the standard American diet, your fiber will at least double by adding this single habit. The USRDA is 30 grams, though government standards are rather unambitious, politically motivated, lowest-common-denominator standards. You

actually need 50–70 grams. Don't be daunted by those fig-
ures. Make a gradual increase but, above all, don't stay at the
typical American's 10–15 grams per day, where your disease
risk is very high.

5

Which Greens
and Why?

The two charts on the following pages detail the wide variety
of nutrient content in greens. They show you why primates in
the wild don't just eat one green food—they eat the biggest
variety available to them. We should do the same with our
smoothies and salads.

These greens may not currently be in your diet but they
should be. Now, with green smoothies, they're easy. No leafy
green is identical, in terms of taste or nutrition, so be bold and
try them all when they're in season and affordable.

Arugula

I'm addicted to this peppery cruciferous green; my mouth literally waters when I think of it. It's very tender and mustardy,
peppery, and nutty. It's most similar to watercress, less strongly
flavored than turnip, dandelion, and mustard greens, which I
consider the most bitter. It's eaten often in Italy, where it

grows wild. It's extremely high in calcium, vitamin C, and beta-carotene. It's beautiful in salads, and also used in Arugula Arame Attack.

Beet greens

One reason I love to grow beets in my garden is that not only do I adore the root vegetable, but it's a bonus food because of what grows above ground and how perfect the leaves and stalks are in green smoothies. Too many people throw this valuable food away because they don't know what to do with it, or they don't even know if it's edible. You can "thin" the stalks while allowing the beets to continue to grow underground. Just cut one or two of the biggest leaves off, close to the ground. They're not bitter and very robust; they'll remind you of the beet itself, in the green form. They're very high in iron, calcium, and vitamin C. See Sweet Beet Slam for a way to use your beet greens.

Bok choy

I buy bok choy and baby bok choy, as well as the leafy green yu choy, frequently and inexpensively at a little Asian market near my home. They're mild in flavor and high in water content. Boy choy is a cruciferous vegetable like broccoli, protecting you from cancer with a compound called sulfurophane, plus it contains lots of vitamins C and A. Try Cabbage Cool-Aid or Asian Green Smoothie to use your bok choy.

Percentage of USRDA of minerals found in one cooked cup, except romaine (2 raw cups) and fennel (1 raw cup). The – symbol indicates unknown or negligible.

GREEN	Protein grams	Calcium	Iron	Magnesium	Phosphorus	Potassium	Zinc	Copper	Manganese	Selenium
Purslane	1.7 g	9%	15%	19%	4%	16%	1%	7%	18%	1%
Kale	2.5 g	9%	7%	6%	4%	9%	–	10%	27%	–
Dandelion greens	2.1 g	15%	10%	6%	4%	7%	2%	6%	12%	–
Collard greens	2.1 g	23%	5%	8%	5%	14%	5%	–	54%	–
Spinach	5.35 g	25%	36%	39%	10%	24%	9%	16%	84%	4%
Chard	3.3 g	10%	22%	38%	6%	27%	4%	15%	29%	–
Fennel	–	4%	4%	4%	4%	10%	–	3%	8%	–
Turnip greens	1.6 g	20%	6%	8%	4%	8%	–	18%	25%	–
Mustard greens	3.2 g	10%	5%	5%	6%	8%	–	6%	19%	–
Romaine	1.8 g	4%	7%	–	5%	9%	–	–	36%	–
Beet greens	3.7 g	16%	15%	24%	6%	37%	5%	18%	37%	2%

Percentage of USRDA of vitamins found in one cooked cup, except romaine (2 raw cups) and fennel (1 raw cup). The − symbol indicates unknown or negligible.

GREEN	Fiber	Folate	Riboflavin B2	Pantothenic Acid B5	Niacin B3	Thiamine B1	Vita A	Vita B6	Vita C	Vita E	Vita K
Purslane	−	3%	6%	−	3%	2%	43%	4%	20%	−	−
Kale	2.6 g	4%	5%	−	3%	5%	192%	9%	89%	6%	1328%
Dandelion greens	−	3%	11%	1%	3%	9%	144%	8%	32%	13%	724%
Collard greens	5.3 g	44%	12%	4%	6%	5%	119%	12%	57%	8%	880%
Spinach	4.3 g	66%	25%	−	4%	11%	295%	22%	29%	9%	1110%
Chard	3.7 g	4%	9%	3%	3%	−	110%	8%	53%	17%	716%
Fennel	2.7 g	6%	−	−	3%	−	−	−	17%	−	−
Turnip greens	−	43%	6%	−	3%	4%	85%	7%	59%	14%	524%
Mustard greens	2.8 g	56%	5%	−	3%	4%	85%	7%	59%	14%	524%
Romaine	1.9 g	38%	7%	−	3%	7%	58%	3%	45%	−	144%
Beet greens	4.2 g	5%	24%	5%	4%	11%	220%	10%	60%	13%	871%

Broccoli rabe

You can get this leafy green, with its stalks, leaves, and little florets, in Italian or Asian markets, and while it's related to broccoli, it isn't part of the broccoli plant. It's fairly bitter, so use small amounts of it in your green smoothie until you taste it to see if it's safe to add more. It's cruciferous like broccoli, which makes it a food with the highest class of cancer-fighting compounds. You can use this ingredient in Broccoli Blitz. Also try baby broccoli (kind of a hybrid between broccoli florets and a leafy green) and the greens on top of the root vegetable kohlrabi, when you can get them.

Cabbage

You have many varieties to choose from, with types from all over the world. Many of my favorites, including baby bok choy, are found in Asian markets and not your typical American market. The sulfurophane in these cruciferous vegetables are well documented to fight cancerous tumor formation and growth. Use green cabbage, red (or purple) cabbage, or "non-head" cabbages such as savoy or black cabbage. Recipes in this book calling for cabbage include Beet Blast, Melon-Seed Melange, Cabbage Cool-Aid, Red Raspberry Radicchio, Asian Green Smoothie, and Big Black Cabbage Cocktail.

Chard

I love chard, my favorite green to grow in my garden. It's prolific and it's a perennial, so if you leave it overwintered, you'll have some first thing in the spring as well. Rainbow chard is so gorgeous in the garden, and you can "cut and come again" throughout its long growing season. Long after spinach has bolted, chard plants are heavy producers and big contributors to my green smoothies through the summer and fall. You have a variety to choose from, including green/white Swiss chard with wide, celery-like ribs, red chard, and highly colorful rainbow chard. The chard family is very high in vitamins A and C. Use chard in One Really Grape Smoothie, Cranapple Yogurt Crave, Kiwi Banana Crush, and Pear Date Purée.

Collard greens

People think collards are for Southerners to fry in bacon fat. In a smoothie, you can tap the incredible nutrition of this powerhouse without destroying nutrients by cooking it or adding fat. Its nutrient profile is even better than broccoli and spinach, with lots of B vitamins, calcium, vitamin C, and beta-carotene. Feel free to use the long stalks in smoothies for a big contribution of fiber to your diet. Collards are mild flavored and a staple in smoothies at my house, as you can tell by the many recipes you'll find collards in. Check out these recipes toward the end of this book: Laura's No-Fruit Green Smoothie, Southern Turnip-Collard Watermelon Cooler, Gobs of Goji, Cranapple Yogurt Crave, Red Leaf Rocks, Aloe and Apple, and Latin Green Smoothie.

Dandelion greens

You dig them out of your yard, even hate them, but did you know they're a nutritional boon for your green smoothies? Pick them in unsprayed fields, not by a roadway, and add smaller amounts to your smoothie, as dandelion greens can be bitter, especially if picked after the plant blooms. The recipes featuring this "free" delicacy at the end of the book are Sodium Dandelion Blast and Dandelion Delight.

Kale

Kale has standout nutritional properties as a cruciferous vegetable related to broccoli, with incredibly high fiber, as well as lots of calcium and vitamins A and C. It usually makes "top ten" lists for power foods. Think of it as dragging your entire gastrointestinal tract, mopping up and carrying out toxic, diseased cells. It's a great smoothie ingredient and is quite mild tasting. You'll enjoy trying all the varieties: black (lacinato), curly (dinosaur), Red Russian, Italian, and flowering kale. Try these recipes to use your entire leaves and stalks of organic kale: Laura's No-Fruit Green Smoothie, Kale Tangelo Tonic, Black Kale Blackberry Brew, Late-Summer Apricot Watercress Divine, Pomegranate Potion, Gobs of Goji, Red Brussels, and Green Chocolate Cooler.

Lettuce and salad greens

Lettuces may include romaine, red and green leaf lettuce, Boston/Bibb, oakleaf, iceberg, chickweed, miner's lettuce, and more—almost too many varieties to mention. All are good, though iceberg lettuce is lower in nutrition, and I'd recommend looking for greener, more colorful options since, generally speaking, the deeper the green, the higher the nutrition. Also consider the hardier and more pungent varieties of salad greens like arugula, watercress, mache, mizuna, frisée, and radicchio. *Mesclun* is the word for a mixture of seedling or baby lettuces and greens. The nutritional profiles vary significantly, but a wide variety is key. The lettuces are soft and make for a very smooth blended drink. Many recipes in this book call for lettuces, including Red Leaf Rocks, Glorious Green Leaf Butterhead Brew, Green Chocolate Cooler, and Chia Choice.

Mustard greens

This is a green that you'll likely either love or hate. I love it because it has some qualities of mustard, kind of a tangy kick. Don't use too much of it in your green smoothie, but it's another way to get variety of nutrition and taste. Try out Mustard Green Mambo in the recipes found in this book.

Spinach

Spinach is so versatile that it's in most of my green smoothies. It's mild tasting and smooth when you blend it, and, therefore, it's my first choice for converting people, especially children, to a green smoothie habit. It's over 42 percent protein, and a serving a day provides your daily requirement for folic acid, plus plenty of iron and vitamins A, C, and E. It's also easy to find all year round and inexpensive in 40-ounce bags at Costco, so as you undertake your new habit, always be aware of the spinach you have on hand so you know whether or not to stock up each time you stop at a grocery store. Because it's high in oxalic acid, which can bind calcium and iron, use a variety of greens rather than spinach only. However, one research study says that when foods containing oxalates are blended, it renders the oxalates harmless. I've eaten handfuls of spinach daily for 15 years without any ill health effects. Many of the recipes at the end of this book use spinach, often in combination with another stronger-tasting green.

Turnip greens

Turnip greens are something you'll like if you like turnips. Like mustard greens, they have a kick but are not nearly as spicy as mustard greens. They're higher than most other greens in calcium, and they're also rich in vitamins A and E, as well as potassium and iron. I love using the tender greens from baby turnips I get in my Community Supported Agriculture share. Try the Southern Turnip-Collard Watermelon Cooler recipe in this book to use your turnip greens.

Watercress

Watercress grows wild and, like most wild plants, outshines the cultivated plants for nutrition: it has as much vitamin A as a carrot and triple the calcium of spinach. It's also high in vitamin C and several of the B vitamins. It's spicy and peppery, so use a bunch in your green smoothie but balance it with some spinach or mild green like collards or chard. Try Watercress Avocado Dream or Late-Summer Apricot Watercress Divine in this book's recipes.

Wild greens

The weeds that grow in your backyard can be a highly nutritious, fun, and, best of all, free source of green smoothie ingredients. You can google photos of these plants that are edible and fair game in your blender: chickweed, a few varieties of lambsquarter, purslane, thistle (I find this to tickle the throats of some who drink it, so use it cautiously at first), curled dock, dandelion greens, morning glory, and amaranth. You can take a nature walk with a plant expert to find these weeds, or purchase one of several books available, if googling for photos doesn't educate you well enough. Just avoid picking weeds next to exhaust-choked roads or fields that have been sprayed or are next to fields that are sprayed. Try Robyn's Green Smoothie Template Recipe or Everything + the Kitchen Sink Garden Smoothie recipe in this book to use any edible weeds you can find!

6

Why Green Smoothies?

Smoothies, big deal, you say. I certainly didn't invent the concept. You've had them before. But, in the past, you've thought of them as a frozen-fruit treat. The whole point with green smoothies is to maximize the greens, to add foods to your concoctions that you know are good for you but you perhaps rarely eat. If you need to, start with more fruit and less greens, but work your way up to the maximum green content. Remember, that's the point.

The benefits are so enormous that I've outlined them here, Letterman-style (but in no particular order), as the Top Ten reasons you should consider this ten-minutes-daily lifestyle change.

1. You're going to eat amazingly nutritious green food you haven't been eating, maybe ever.

When was the last time you ate a big plate of plain collards, chard, carrot tops, and celery? Have you ever? Especially plain without gobs of ranch dressing? Mustard greens, arugula, turnip greens, dandelion greens, beet greens, and chard don't end up in too many salads, even for the most health conscious among us. Even most raw foodists are deficient in greens.

Just the time to chew the above-described plate of greens would take 30 minutes—and add chopping time to that. But those items and more will be in your green smoothies every day.

I drink a quart, and my kids drink a pint, every day. You can make the smoothies ahead of time and stick them in the fridge for a later meal or snack. You can store them for up to 48 hours—just shake very well before drinking.

2. You don't have to use high-fat, chemical-laden salad dressings to "get it down."

Another benefit of a smoothie versus a salad is that all green smoothie ingredients are whole plant foods, with low calories and little or no added fat. Any fat you do add will be from high-quality, plant-based sources. Many people are not aware that salad dressings you purchase in the store are full of toxic chemicals like the deadly excitotoxin monosodium glutamate or MSG (which goes by many names you may not recognize on a label); the very worst refined sweetener, high-fructose corn syrup; refined salt; and rancid, refined oils like soybean and other vegetable oils. Many salads end up being rather high in calories and having some of the same ingredients in junk foods. Infamously, McDonald's salads sometimes are as high in calories as their other meals.

3. You will be living the way God or Nature has always intended you to eat, similar to the way animals related to humans eat.

Victoria Boutenko studied the dietary habits of our closest relatives, large primates. Because we share 99.4 percent of our

DNA with our cousins, the primates, we'd do well to observe what they do in nature, driven by instinct. (Disclaimer: This is not an endorsement of evolutionary theory or any disavowal of the idea that God created the world. It's simply relating the science of our similarity to primates.)

Of course, primates are largely vegetarian and eat a diet of primarily greens. Gorillas don't eat a whole tree in a day; rather, they eat a little every day of a wide variety of greens. In their natural environment, eating what instinct tells them to, they experience little or no degenerative disease. We've lost our instincts to eat whole plant foods since we've been eating unnatural processed foods for several generations and are heavily influenced by the chemical disruptors in those foods that make us crave the wrong foods and find the right foods offensive, tedious to eat, or boring. (Fortunately, even a short period of time eliminating those foods often allows us to return to our original cravings.)

4. A high-power blender breaks down walls of cellulose better than your teeth can, making nutrition immediately available and predigested.

Boutenko recommends you try an experiment of chewing your salad up: right before you would normally swallow it, spit it out and look at it. To be digestible, it needs to be fully broken down into the tiniest particles—"creamed" like wide-palate primates with strong jaws are able to do easily, without any observable "chunks" of green.

You're likely to see a mouthful of torn-up greens, nowhere near "creamed." That's because over the past few generations, our palates have narrowed (thus the meteoric rise in ortho-dontic work—more and more orthodontists are widening children's palates). Our jaws have weakened. We're no longer capable of breaking down through mastication the most important foods in our diet, greens.

The problem is, we've devolved as a species as a result of eating an increasingly soft-food (processed) diet the past few generations. Parents in today's generation protect their children from having to chew much of anything. Many cut the peel off their children's apples, even after all the children's teeth have come in. Some of my friends even cut the crusts off their children's white-bread sandwiches!

Plant fiber is completely missing from the diets of modern children as their muscles are developing. An open-minded child willing to eat a salad is likely to barely chew it before swallowing, and while the insoluble fiber is still beneficial, no doubt, the body simply cannot break down and utilize the nutrition in the greens without being fully chewed.

Blended greens have been shown to increase nutrient absorption. Gray hair, for instance, is a sign of mineral deficiency. Ann Wigmore, the wheatgrass juice pioneer, famously regained her hair color by eating blended greens.

Maybe you can't back up "devolution" of the jaw. But the good news is that while I still highly recommend salads, and chewing them well, a high-power blender "creams" the greens—i.e., predigests them—for you. It breaks them down and actually crushes the cell walls, making nutrients highly bioavailable when eaten right after processing in your blender. The only thing you need to do with your green smoothie is "chew" it fully in your mouth (even though it's smooth and liquified) to add the important digestive juices and enzymes from saliva to your food before it goes to the stomach.

5. Green smoothie prep is the highest-impact task you can undertake in your kitchen: the highest and best use of your time.

Green smoothie preparation is the biggest "bang for the buck" and the biggest "return on investment" of your time spent in food preparation. The first time I measured, I couldn't believe how much green food a quart of smoothie has in it: 15 full servings of raw greens and fruit and 12 or more grams of fiber (depending on ingredients), even with 25 percent of the smoothie being water. That's 150 percent of the USRDA's suggested fruit and vegetable intake for an entire day. (I believe that their requirements are very low and highly influenced by the processed-food and meat and dairy industries.) You'll see when you make your first smoothie that mountains of greens blend down to a very compact, drinkable, nutritional package.

Salads involve chopping. Green smoothies made in a high-power blender don't. Raw-food recipes involve peeling, cutting, arranging, and, often, many steps. Green smoothies involve throwing everything in the fridge in a blender and pouring it out into a jar. It just couldn't be simpler. You don't have to be a gourmet, and even people who don't cook at all can do it easily.

I once taught green smoothies to a single father I was dating. He worked heavy hours and lived in a city where he had custody of his active, athletic boys, with no family in the area to help with childcare. He was the quintessential overworked parent in America whose every minute is measured in terms of impact. (Actually, he's Australian, but they have the same issues there that Americans do!) He said to me, "I am the stereotype of the person who needs your program. And, *this* thing, I can do!" His boys drank their first green smoothie and ran out into the yard, doing cartwheels and running in circles, yelling, "My eyesight's getting better! I can feel it!" We didn't continue dating, but he did continue making green smoothies and participated in the research at the end of this book.

6. You get more live enzymes in blended green drinks than in any other food.

Drinking a quart a day of green smoothie addresses what I believe is the number-one deficit in the American diet: *lack of enzymes*. Enzymes are catalysts in all bodily functions, including digestion. Digestive enzymes break down food for storage, and while your body's organs can produce the needed digestive enzymes, those organs typically become exhausted in anyone eating a typical Western diet of dead, processed foods. You have, at best, according to most estimates, about 30 years' worth of enzyme-production capacity. Eating raw foods, particularly leafy greens that have intact enzymes, gives you energy that does not deplete your limited enzymatic capacity. (And I'm not including iceberg lettuce in the category of "leafy greens," because it's a low-nutrition food relative to other lettuces and is not easily digested by humans, so I suggest spending your food dollars on other greens for your smoothies.)

Enzymes are retained when foods are never heated above 116 degrees—and to be safe, I try to stay at 105 degrees or lower when dehydrating or blending foods. Drinking a quart of green smoothie daily will go a long way in providing your body the enzymes it needs to digest other cooked food.

Dr. Edward Howell spent 20 years writing *Enzyme Nutrition: The Food Enzyme Concept* after studying enzymes for several decades of his medical career. We're eating so much dead food, which we're not designed to do, and it's leading to all the degenerative diseases of our day—autoimmune, cancer, heart problems, and more. Howell says that disease started when man discovered fire and began killing food enzymes with it.

The critical law of biology that Howell explains is that when we require our body to manufacture enzymes to simply digest our food, by eating food without its own enzymes, we are robbing more important needs for enzyme activity in metabolic processes. That's every single transaction that takes place in every organ. And the result of stealing enzymes from where they belong is cell damage, burnout, aging—and, ultimately, early death. This phenomenon of burning out our natural resources manifests itself as disease. All of these tragedies are entirely preventable if we eat food containing enzymes.

Howell outlines three types of enzymes we need: *digestive* enzymes, which digest food, *metabolic* enzymes, which run every function of our bodies, and *food* enzymes from raw foods, which start the digestive process. So what enzymes are involved in digestion?

Amylase digests carbohydrates, and is concentrated in saliva. *Protease* digests proteins, found in concentration in the stomach. *Lipase* digests fats and is manufactured by the pancreas (along with additional amounts of amylase and protease).

Exogenous food enzymes (from the outside, from raw food or enzyme supplements) are critical because you need your *endogenous* enzyme activity (manufactured by the pancreas) to be allocated to metabolic processes. When your body has to produce concentrated digestive enzymes because your food didn't arrive with its own live enzymes, you're guilty of forcing your precious enzyme activity to do the labor of digestion while also expecting it to metabolize well. Results include all the disease effects of using up limited resources in the wrong places.

What most of us learned in biology classes when we were young isn't totally accurate. That is, we were taught that the 3,000 enzymes discovered (and likely many more undiscovered) are catalysts, the sparks needed for every action and reaction in the body. They're, in fact, catalysts—used in chemical activities (in this case, in living beings). But that doesn't tell the whole story because that's not all enzymes are. They have more *biological* functions beyond the neutral chemical-catalyst role. They contain proteins, and some contain vitamins. Plus, they do wear out, and are routinely flushed out by the organs of elimination. We make a truly fatal mistake believing that we can waste them indiscriminately.

The best way to stay youthful and avoid drawing on our precious enzyme-manufacturing resources is through the highest consumption possible of raw plant food, especially greens, at every meal. Greens are the highest-enzyme foods you can possibly eat.

7. Smoothies retain all the fiber in the plant, without massive cleanup, compared to juicing.

Many of us "health nuts" have a Champion, Jack LaLanne, or Omega juicer collecting dust in a back cupboard and making us feel guilty. We've juiced in fits and starts. These outdated kitchen tools make a huge mess and cost us a lot of time to clean up and put away the many breakable parts, so I've found in informal polling that no one really makes a habit of juicing, daily, long term, even though we may like the health benefits. A high-power blender allows you to leverage all the benefits of many plant foods without throwing away most of the plant. Plus, as nutritious as a glass of carrot juice is, it contains the sugar of several carrots without the fiber, so there is nothing to help slow the absorption of sugar into the bloodstream.

Green smoothies are packed with insoluble plant fiber. Insoluble plant fiber is the best broom: It cleans out the 30-plus feet of your entire digestive tract. Think of your greens as a little muscle-bound green guy: He can carry out of your body several times more than his own body weight in toxic compounds that arrived through food, air, water, and stress. No spoonful of chemically reduced Metamucil can do what the natural fiber in plants can do. (In fact, Metamucil can be a colon irritant.)

After the number-one deficit described above, live enzymes, perfectly addressed by green smoothies, the number-two deficit in the Western diet is *lack of overall plant fiber in the diet*. Because fiber is removed from refined foods, Americans eat an average of only 11–14 grams per day (you get that much or more in your green smoothie alone), and the USRDA recommendation is 25–30 grams.

I strongly recommend that at least 40–50 grams is ideal. A chimpanzee in the wild (left to his own devices to choose his diet) eats 300 grams per day! As with many other things, the FDA and USDA cave to meat and dairy interests and water down the truth to appease those industries and avoid overwhelming "middle America." Of course, drinking a quart of green smoothie daily addresses this critical issue of insufficient plant fiber, too.

Fiber lowers blood cholesterol level and stabilizes blood sugar. It prevents hemorrhoids and constipation and every disease of the colon. Eating plenty of plant fiber is the best and, really, only way to avoid colon cancer, a leading cause of death and misery in the U.S. Insoluble plant fiber, while not digested, is critical in removing toxins, including metals, from

the body. It's found abundantly in greens, as well as vegetables, beans, whole grains, legumes, nuts, and seeds.

8. Green smoothies are fast to prepare and fast to eat.

I love that green smoothies are "fast food" that is healthful,
since those two conditions don't coincide in the same food
very often. I do love salads for sit-down meals, to further aug-
ment consumption of greens and vegetables. But, unlike a
salad, I can make a green smoothie the night before and put it
in a quart jar in the fridge. When I leave for work, I grab the
smoothie, a straw, and a napkin and put them in an insulated
lunchbox with a re-freezable coolant. Your co-workers will
definitely say, "*What is that?!*" if you drink it openly like I do,
always hoping for a convert. (If you're shy, you can always
hide with a thermos.) But if you respond with enthusiasm and
a testimonial about the health benefits you've experienced,
some of them will ask you later how to make it. (I've been
known to thrust my green smoothie at random strangers with
an extra straw and say, "Try it!")

Take one to work the next day for your co-worker, and
spread the word as your good deed for the day. Pretty soon
your whole office will be converted. People love a live demo,
if you're willing to bring your high-power blender and greens
to work—but I've given very detailed instructions in my "template recipe," and you can also guide others to my three-
minute green smoothie demo on GreenSmoothieGirl. com and
YouTube. (Also see my more advanced "green smoothie 2.0"
demo [part 1 and 2] showing all the superfoods you can add,
as well as a two-part video of me in the grocery store choosing
greens and giving you tips on that subject.)

9. You have a lower impact on the environment and you're eating lower on the food chain.

We first undertake a habit like this because of the personal gain, but what a fantastic side benefit that we benefit the environment as well. When you eat plant food, you're requiring one-twentieth the resources of the earth, in terms of acreage and water, as you do when you eat the same quantity of food in the form of beef. Further, all the scraps can go into a compost pile to become fertilizer for even more plant food later on.

If you don't garden, you can still toss your scraps on the ground outside. Even if they go to the landfill, they decompose quickly, unlike boxes and plastic used for packaged foods that may never decompose. Consider that every bit of green smoothie you consume is that much of some other food you didn't eat. Your carbon footprint is smaller with every green smoothie you drink.

And no animals have to die or be miserably penned up in a too-small stall or cage to satisfy your caloric needs today.

10. Green smoothies actually taste good—almost anyone will drink them, including the vegetable-phobic and the very young!

Green smoothies are a health food that you can actually look forward to. I feel the same way about a day without a green smoothie as I do a day without breaking a sweat, or a day without praying. Something is missing, and my day just doesn't go as well.

I honestly look forward to my smoothie every day. Now, I'll admit, sometimes I make a smoothie that doesn't taste great—I'm always pushing the outer limits of the greens-to-fruit ratio. But, most of the time, it really does taste good (when I make that a priority), and while green blended drinks are an acquired taste for some, they really can be very pleasant to drink. Most reported in Boutenko's small Roseburg study that they wished they had *more* than a quart a day. I've never met a child who won't drink one, especially if you add more fruit and make sure the color isn't actually green. There's simply no better way to "hide" nutrition from young and picky eaters.

7

How Green Smoothies Change Lives

I polled GreenSmoothieGirl.com readers to gather data about what difference, if any, their green-smoothie habit made in their lives, and I was interested in health benefits as well as cleansing reactions (or challenges). I've found that when I show people what a high-impact habit this is, and I assign them the mission of converting others, they undertake that challenge with enthusiasm. So I wondered whether my quest is going quantum, and I polled my readers about whether they've been evangelizing for green smoothies. This research is ongoing, so please fill out the questionnaire at GreenSmoothie Girl.com after you've been drinking green smoothies for at least one month.

Before I share the data with you from 175 respondents who had been drinking green smoothies for at least 30 days, at least a pint three times a week, here is the questionnaire:

GREEN SMOOTHIE QUESTIONNAIRE

Have you found that green smoothies have noticeably improved your health or quality of life?   Yes   /   No

What health benefits have you noticed from drinking green smoothies? (Check all that apply.)

☐ Improved digestion: more regular and/or complete bowel movements, no straining, soft/formed stool, etc.

☐ Weight loss

☐ More energy

☐ Improved sleep: need less of it, decreased insomnia, more alert in the mornings, etc.

☐ Decreased cravings for sweets and processed foods

☐ Fingernails: faster growth and/or stronger nails

☐ Decrease in PMS symptoms

☐ Improved libido (sex drive)

☐ Positive, stable mood

☐ Less stressed out

☐ Blood sugar stabilization

☐ Increased desire to exercise

☐ Improvement in skin tone, fewer blemishes

☐ People telling me I look better

☐ Hair: shinier, and/or dandruff gone

☐ Other: _____

If you have lost weight, how many pounds have you lost? _____ [fill in the blank]

Did you have any uncomfortable cleansing reactions as you began drinking green smoothies?   Yes   /   No

If so, what were they?

_____ [fill in the blank]

Have you seen any chronic or degenerative conditions improve or go away? If so, please explain:

_____

_____

Have you felt so positively about your green smoothie conversion that you've converted anyone else?   Yes   /   No

Research Results

The results of my poll of 175 green-smoothie drinkers yielded some interesting results that suggest quite definitively that it's a ten-minute habit worth adopting! To participate in the questionnaire, one had to be drinking green smoothies for at least 30 days, a pint a day for at least three days a week. Many were drinking more, up to my recommended quart daily.

The vast majority, or 95.4 percent, said green smoothies noticeably improved their health or quality of life. Very exciting to me is the fact that 84 percent of those drinking green smoothies are so enthusiastic about the positive health benefits that they've told others about or taught them the habit!

These are the positive health effects people experience, listed in order of their frequency among the research respondents:

- 85 percent experience *more energy*.
- 79.5 percent experience *improved digestion* (more regular and/or complete bowel movements, no straining, soft/formed stool, etc.).
- 65 percent experience *fewer cravings* for sweets and processed foods.
- 54 percent experience a *more positive, stable mood*.
- 50 percent experience an *improvement in skin tone*, or fewer blemishes.
- 50 percent experience *weight loss*. The average reported pounds lost was 18.25 pounds!

(Keep in mind when considering this very impressive statistic that some of the respondents had been drinking green smoothies only 30 days, and some of them did not have any weight to lose. But 87 out of 175 respondents reported a total of over 1,500 pounds of weight lost!)

- 46.3 percent experience an *increased desire to exercise*.

- 45 percent experience *improved sleep* (need less of it, decreased insomnia, more alert in the mornings, etc.).
- 44 percent feel *less stressed out.*
- 39 percent experience *blood sugar stabilization.*
- 37 percent say their *fingernails are stronger or grow faster.*
- 36 percent experience people telling them they *look better.*
- 27.5 percent say their *hair is shinier* or their dandruff gone.
- 22 percent experience a *decrease in PMS symptoms.* (Consider that some of the respondents in the survey are not females of menstruating age.)
- 20 percent report an *improved sex drive.*

Other positive health benefits reported by survey respondents include:

- 8 people said: Arthritis symptoms/pain gone or reduced
- 3 people said: Hyperthyroid condition improved (reduced or gone off meds)
- 2 people said: Seasonal allergies gone or decreased
- 3 people said: Reduced asthma symptoms
- 2 people said: Migraines gone or reduced by 80 percent
- 2 people said: Acne improved or gone
- 2 people said: Eczema or dry skin cleared
- 2 people said: Gray hair returned to original color
- 2 people said: Gallstones gone
- 2 people said: Decreased blood pressure
- No more hypertension
- Was able to go off cholesterol meds
- Was able to go off Prilosec
- Haven't gotten sick in a year like I always do

- Moles disappeared
- Deep facial wrinkles "barely noticeable"
- Less nasal congestion
- Lump on leg getting smaller
- Liver spots fading
- Tendonitis gone
- Muscle soreness gone
- Fibromyalgia symptoms disappearing
- Hypoglycemia improved
- No more bloating, gas, indigestion, constipation
- Avoided a hysterectomy; 2 people said lifelong menstrual problems returned to normal
- Hot flashes stopped
- No more aching muscles after hard workouts
- No more reflux/nausea after eating
- No more insomnia
- Easier to breastfeed
- Don't sunburn anymore
- Depression symptoms gone
- Lifelong bad breath gone in two weeks
- Ended coffee addiction
- More alkaline body pH
- Just feel better

Only 18.3 percent had uncomfortable, short-term cleansing reactions. The following symptoms were reported:

- Headaches
- Diarrhea
- Bloating
- Cramps
- Vertigo
- Fainting
- Skin breakouts
- Nausea
- Intestinal gas
- Constipation
- Dizziness
- Lethargy or weakness

- Runny nose
- Cold/virus
- Depression
- Mucus in the back of the throat
- Liver pain/liver cleansing
- Mood swings
- Emotional crisis

The risks of a new green-smoothie habit are limited to an 18.3 percent chance of short-term discomfort. The top six benefits that people experience when starting a green smoothie habit are, in order, more energy, improved digestion, fewer cravings for sweets and processed food, a more positive/stable mood, improved skin, and weight loss.

The testimonials submitted with this data are inspiring and are included at the end of this book. It's hard to look at this data without being compelled to give green smoothies a try!

8

Your First
Challenge:
A Quart a Day

So, you say, I'm sold! How much should I drink, then?

You may want to work your way up from a lesser amount, but a great goal is to have a quart a day. Using Robyn's Green Smoothie Template Recipe (page 144) that appears first in this book's recipe section, a quart is 15 servings of greens and fruit based on the U.S. Recommended Daily Allowances serving sizes! For most people, that's 750–1,500 percent more vegetables and fruits than they're currently getting.

Please note that I think the USRDA serving sizes are shockingly small. A better target is 20–25 servings daily of those serving sizes, and my family achieves that higher goal virtually every day without difficulty, just by making fruits and vegetables the crux of our diet, eating till we're satisfied, and leaving refined foods out of the menu. For children, try to achieve a goal of a pint a day (or less for babies and toddlers). That's 7.5 adult USRDA servings of raw plant food.

You won't "overdose" on green smoothies unless you have some very rare conditions where excessive vitamin K or another nutrient must be avoided. Sometimes I "detox" by eating nothing but blended drinks for a day or even a few days. One woman chronicled months of how she lost over 100 pounds consuming nothing at all except green smoothies over five months in an online blog.

You may, if you haven't been on a highly plant-based diet for a while, experience diarrhea or other cleansing reactions as discussed further on in this book. My research, summarized later in this book, indicates that 18.5 percent of green smoothie newbies have "cleansing reactions." If you're in that number, those reactions are temporary, a manifestation of your body recognizing good building and cleansing materials coming in, and an opportunity to throw out diseased, toxic, waste materials.

Sometimes when our tired, clogged, overworked organs begin receiving excellent nutrition, they can become overwhelmed, and uncomfortable reactions result. Those reactions rarely last longer than two weeks and are usually, in fact, much shorter in duration. They commonly include headaches, digestive disturbances, skin breakouts or rashes, a feeling of sluggishness, sleep problems, or other symptoms. Be patient with your body and don't let a little discomfort allow you to quit the path.

What Tools Do I Need?

Only two blenders on the market are worth your money: Vita-Mix and Blendtec. I have owned both for years. They're not really blenders—they're really called whole-food machines because they're so competent and have so many uses that a regular blender cannot compete with. All other blenders burn up, and not only will you be frustrated by having to buy blender after blender when they do, but you'll also have to leave out hard-core ingredients, like big frozen strawberries and the stems of greens. You save money in the long run and have better blended drinks if you invest in the right machine the first time.

I use my turbo blenders several times a day, seven days a week. I often say when I teach classes that it's the best thing I own. People think I mean it's the best thing I own in my kitchen but, actually, it's the best thing I own, period. It's so much more than a blender because it grinds wheat or flaxseed or coffee, it makes perfect soups without a stove, it crushes ice, and it makes frozen desserts, salad dressings, sauces, and more.

The two brands cost the same—and I'll leave any other competition out of the comparison because these two big guys, Vita-Mix and Blendtec, are the best. (I also own a Bosch blender and some others, but they don't even belong in the comparison.)

This is my review of the strengths of both machines:

BLENDTEC

1. Blendtec's motor is 3 horsepower, compared to Vita-Mix's 2.5. That's more horsepower to blend even big frozen chunks of fruit and the most fibrous greens.

2. Blendtec is the smarter machine, with 17 settings for blending really anything. The smoothie setting alternates high and low to pull greens down centrifugally into the "blending vortex" during the slow cycles. That way you don't have to muscle your greens down with a tamper.

3. Blendtec has a lifetime warranty on the blade so you don't have to worry about it getting dull.

4. Blendtec's product is smaller and fits under standard countertops (unlike Vita-Mix, which does not fit, so you have to remove the container). I take mine to hotel rooms so my family's nutrition doesn't suffer on the road—it fits neatly in a suitcase.

5. Blendtec has the square jar design that's both easier to pour from and wider. The Vita-Mix is deeper and narrow, and you have to scrape stuff out of the bottom, so food is wasted.

6. With Blendtec, you don't have to buy a second container with a special blade for dry ingredients. (That costs you an extra $80 with the Vita-Mix.) Thus, you can blend wheat into flour without purchasing an additional appliance.

VITAMIX

1. The machine has the better warranty and the company has outstanding customer service.

2. I like the tamper tool for blending very thick concoctions more easily, through a hole in the top of the lid, using a little muscle power. (You can get a free tamper for the Blendtec online, but the company does not approve of its use.)

3. The canister that comes with the Vita-Mix is bigger (96-ounce) than Blentec's. (You can buy an extra canister for the Blendtec.)

Nobody who is serious about raw, whole-food nutrition (especially getting greens into the diet) should be without a Blendtec or Vita-Mix machine. I believe outstanding nutrition is so much easier to achieve with a turbo blender. It's the very first thing I ask of my readers in *12 Steps to Whole Foods*. It's a significant investment at approximately $400, but you'll never be sorry you made it.

If you have a family, I recommend ordering the larger (96-ounce) blender container if you get a Blendtec. This way you can maximize a single batch, to have a quart for three people (or a quart for you and a pint each for four children, for instance). If you're single or have no children, and/or if you're very busy and want to cut your prep time in half, this also allows you to make twice as much as you need and refrigerate the remainder.

Mark the cups on a turbo blender container all the way to the top with a permanent marker. Do this by running tap water into the container up to the top line, 4 cups. Then add another cup and mark the water level. Then add another cup and mark that line with your marker. The container that comes with the Vita-Mix and the additional, larger container you can order from Blendtec each allow you to make 96 ounces at a time. This will allow you to make the recipes in this book (yielding three quarts) without having to pour some off, adding fruit, and reblending.

Other items I recommend you have on hand are *quart jars* and *plastic lids* (which can be obtained at any discount retailer like Walmart or Target), and a *bottle washer* to clean them out. Wide-mouth jars are easier to clean than regular jars. Another GreenSmoothieGirl.com reader gave the tip of taking your green smoothie to work inside a plastic bag, just in case the jar breaks. That way you protect your purse, lunch cooler, or duffel bag.

How Do I Drink a Green Smoothie?

Digestion begins in the mouth. So "chew" your smoothie. The one downfall to blended foods is the tendency we have to "slam" them. I admit that sometimes when I make what I call a "hard-core" green smoothie (in other words, lots of weedy or bitter greens and little fruit—or, in other words, a yucky-tasting one), I slam it.

Don't lie awake in bed at night worrying that you didn't "chew" your green smoothie enough. You've done a very good thing to drink a green smoothie, any way that happens, even if it's fed straight from a tube into your stomach. (Still beats a Big Mac and fries, or pretty much anything you were eating before!)

But the best way to drink your green smoothie is, in fact, to "eat" it rather than drink it. That is, even though it's liquid, take the time to "chew" it to stimulate your salivary glands. Slower is better to increase the saliva that begins the digestion enzymatically before your food is in the fundus, or pre-stomach.

9

Your Second Challenge: Be a Green Smoothie Evangelist

I've had many thousands of emails and personal testimonials about green smoothies dramatically changing people's health; I wish I had an exact count! I rarely go to Costco that someone doesn't stop me and say, "Aren't you the GreenSmoothieGirl?" Once a woman proudly pointed out her toddler in the grocery cart, who was sporting a green moustache. Another "stalked" me (her words) several miles to Costco and then walked up to me in the parking lot to say that my program was her cancer battle plan. These experiences make my day.

This is why I spread the gospel of green: I love to hear about how people's health has improved, their outlook on life expanded, their positive energy radiating to others.

And, like all things we find beautiful and life changing, we want to share them with others. If you're a green smoothie convert, your job now is to bless others' lives by telling them how they can spend ten minutes in the kitchen daily and address so many of their nutritional deficits.

Someone in your life is suffering. I don't run down overweight older ladies in the grocery store to tell them they should eat greens, as Victoria Boutenko describes having done in one of her books. (I find this endearing, even while ineffective—the intent and motive is good, while the execution is flawed.) I have learned (as she eventually did, as well) that those who seek are those who learn. While I do not approach people, I do love to give information to those who ask. Those are people ready and willing to learn: the ones who see the difference in your health and appearance, and ask.

As you discuss how excited you are to realize the benefits of getting 15 servings of greens and fruit in your daily diet, you can't help but talk about it at work, at the extended-family get-together, at the gym, at church social events. Tell them how they can learn about green smoothies or invite them over for a demo and taste test at your house. In my survey, I found that the vast majority of those who take the challenge on GreenSmoothieGirl.com to adopt the habit also teach others about it.

You'll have your own story that is similar to mine, and that story does not end with you looking and feeling younger and more positive. It doesn't end with the elimination of chronic health problems for you or even your children. It keeps going and going, with your willingness to promote green smoothies and a plant-based diet and bless others, who then evangelize even more until your sphere of influence is huge! You can make a big impact for good on this world. Not only do you change people's health, but you support growers of plant food, you decrease meat consumption that consumes the world's scarce resources at a frightening pace, and you do great service in a troubled world.

Ten Tips for Helping Kids Go Green

One of the most frequent questions I'm asked is, "How can I get my child to drink green smoothies?" These are my ten suggestions, based on my work with families as well as my own children.

1. Start with mostly fruit smoothies, or naturally sweeten them.

A good ratio to work toward is 50/50: 50 percent greens and 50 percent fruit (over and above the water you start with). In other words, to 3 cups of water, add greens until the blender container is at 6 cups, and then add fruit until the container is at 9 cups. However, for newbies, skeptics, and children, I always suggest starting with more like a 25:75 ratio: 25 percent greens, 75 percent fruit. And use only spinach at first— the vast majority of people won't even notice it in a mostly fruit smoothie.

2. Come up with a great name for your smoothies, and make the whole endeavor fun.

This tip is primarily for parents of young children. And, if you're a parent of a small child, count your blessings, because the younger you make the conversion, the easier it is, generally. I got this idea when I first began making green smoothies in 1994. What I made for ten years is an older, inferior version of canned or frozen pineapple juice, spinach, and alfalfa sprouts. I made my first one on a summer day and was sitting on the front porch watching Kincade, my 18-month-old first child, play. He came up to me and peered in my glass. At that point, it had never occurred to me in my wildest dreams that *he* might drink spinach and sprouts.

He asked, "Whassat?" Thinking quickly (about the possibility of getting him to drink it, and wanting it to be appealing), I said, "Ice cream." He, of course, wanted some. My brain went into overdrive, realizing that I had a possibility to get him to eat something really good for him. But to create scarcity and demand, I said, "This is *Mommy's* ice cream." At this point, he began to beg. I said, "Well. Hmmmm. Okay, I'll give you just a little *taste*." He tasted it and begged for more.

The name morphed quickly into "Green Cream," because that's what he called it. (Apparently he recognized that it was a bit different from real ice cream, but he also connected that I'd originally called it ice cream. Rather brilliant kid, I thought.) My original green drink was half pineapple juice and half greens, whereas now I don't use any juice. But we called it Green Cream until years later when I discovered blended drinks and how much more nutritious, lower in sugar, and higher in fiber they could be.

What does your child love? If he's a rambunctious little boy, call it Power Rangers Super Blaster Formula. If she's a girly girl, call it Pretty Pretty Princess Potion. This makes green smoothies fun. Then, later, if they get bored, change the name.

3. Get your child off sugar.

For adults and children alike, my observation is that virtually everyone who turns up his or her nose at the taste of green smoothies is someone who is addicted to sugar. You don't have to eat tons of refined sugar to be an addict, since it's simply the most addictive substance on the planet. Some studies have documented that it's more powerful and habit-forming than cocaine.

Some very interesting things happen when you quit eating sugar, which I invite you to explore, and I highly recommend putting your children through this withdrawal as well. The first three to four days are grueling. Sugar addicts will experience overwhelming cravings. Most will, in fact, succumb and eat their favorite treats before four days have passed.

But after four days are over (the length can vary but there's a definite period after which cravings decrease dramatically), other foods that didn't taste good before now taste wonderful. The natural, more subtly sweet flavors, such as fruits and dates, are much more appealing.

If you eat a Nestle Toll House cookie on Monday and Tuesday, a naturally sweetened flaxseed cookie isn't that appealing, as one of my *12 Steps to Whole Foods* bloggers on GreenSmoothieGirl.com once noted. But I suggest undergoing withdrawal and trying that same natural treat again—it's an entirely different experience!

Then, once you've gone through that withdrawal for several days (most people don't make it past those worst three to four days), ask yourself something before you eat sugar again. That is, do you really want to bring all the cravings back, along with the attendant blood sugar swings, mood disturbances, energy loss, and headaches?

It's not worth it. (Of course, we've all "fallen off the wagon." But you're beginning to succeed when those falls become less and less frequent.)

Try eliminating all the sugar-sweetened junk from your home. Be prepared for the next several days to be very difficult. Don't be surprised if you have begging, whining, moody children. Realize that this is sugar talking. Do some thinking about what we invite into our homes when we addict our kids to sugar. My own kids do not beg and whine and cajole and cry for treats, ever. When I'm in other parents' homes and see this behavior, I feel sorry for the parents. The kids are addicts and, unlike the adults, they can't get a "fix" whenever they want—they have to beg for their sugar shot. It makes everybody miserable.

In graduate school, studying to be a therapist, I worked for a year on the children's unit of the state mental hospital. I was appalled at the amount of sugar the children were fed. There was a "store" in their in-house school where, for good behavior or grades, they could pick out candy. The cafeteria nutrition was appalling, with plenty of dessert for both lunch and dinner, and the breakfast was a lot of junk, too. And, after school, volunteers always came in and plied the children with cookies and candy. The children were ill constantly in the winter with every virus and bacterial infection; most of them were also overweight.

I went to the director of the children's unit, a psychiatrist, and made my case that the children were being wronged with so much sugar and terrible nutrition. He said to me, "But this is all the love that most of these children get—we can't take that away from them."

We have to break the idea in our own minds, and then not start that awful cycle with our children, thinking of sugar and love as equivalent. When we self-soothe with that deadly chemical, we create a wide variety of consequences, none of them good. When we get off sugar, the best whole foods God put on the planet suddenly taste delicious and desirable.

4. Educate your child about what's in it for her by starting a green smoothie habit.

I have demo videos about some of my ideas (my first homemade tape showing a green smoothie in three minutes, then "Green Smoothie 2.0" about superfoods, and "Educating Kids about Nutrition") that you can find by searching "greensmoothiegirl" on YouTube. (In fact, unrelated to the "Educating Kids" demo, notice that my then-seven-year-old son wandered into the video being made, drinking his green smoothie.)

A basic, simplistic education for kids about *why* we're feeding them this way is mission critical, because we can't force-feed our kids. I once watched one of my good friends completely "lose it" when her son wouldn't eat on a vacation we were on at a lake house. In total frustration, she snapped and began cramming a hot dog down his throat. It was actually one of the funniest things I've ever seen. My friend is a very easygoing parent in general, and I've teased her about that scene for many years. Of course, many parents can relate to stress with issues around kids and eating. (Of course, if you're going to cram food down your own child's throat, may I suggest that you choose something other than a hot dog?)

I talk in a very simplistic way to my young children about nutrition, as I find that it's unwise to not start at a very young age. For instance, children will naturally gravitate toward white bread because it's stark in color and soft. But, with a little explanation, my children understand what the grain itself looks like, because I pull it out of the pantry. I show them that there are three parts to the grain—you can cut the grain in half to show a cross-section, or whiteboard it as I do in my demo video. They learn that the outer part, the *bran*, is what cleans all the garbage out of your guts: it's called fiber. Then, the part barely inside that is called the *germ*, and it has all the vitamins that help you build your bones and have pretty skin. Now, see, inside the wheat berry is snow-white stuff. It's called the *endosperm*, and it's really just the glue that holds it all together. It's not worth much except as glue.

Consequently, my children call white bread "glue." One of them was once overheard holding a bottle of Elmer's Glue and telling her friend that it's the main ingredient in white bread. I obviously had some clarifying to do, and I realized that for younger children, the explanations have to be really clear and simple rather than metaphorical!

The upside has been that over the years of our family being fairly public and fairly well known for our whole-food, plant-based diet, even my children have been instruments of change. They talk about our family's habits and often defend and explain why we eat the way we do. Their friends are curious. Many times parents of their friends have come to me or to my website seeking help and change. I can't say that none of my children has ever been resistant, or that none of my children has ever tired of green smoothies or of explaining our lifestyle to their friends and their friends' parents. All of them are very social and live in the "real world." But even the resistant ones don't like how they feel when they come home from scout camp or girls' camp having missed the benefits of daily green smoothies and lots of nutritious food. Both of my teenagers have walked in the door and, before even completing their hello hug, said to me, "Mom! I need a green smoothie! Seriously, please!"

Explain fiber to even your young children. It's not a nutrient, exactly. It's just scratchy bulk that drags through your many, many feet of intestinal tract. It's like a broom, and it sweeps out all the garbage that accumulates there. Without it, the garbage builds up and builds up until your arteries get clogged and blood can't get through. You have pain and illness, and you gain weight, and your organs like your kidneys and liver can't do their jobs.

That was an example of how I speak to my children. It's different than how I speak to you, or how I write on a scientific topic on my blog. It's plain and simple and uses metaphors they might understand. Green smoothies are a broom. Simple. If you have a child who suffers from constipation, which can be frustrating and painful, you can say that people who drink their green smoothie every day don't get plugged up like he has been. That's because the broom is working all the time. Kids understand this. Over time, what you achieve by educating your children is they *buy-in*. Some children will, even while young, make great choices because that education sinks in. I have kids like that. Others will make poor choices at the neighborhood barbecue, but that doesn't mean your education has fallen on deaf ears. That means they're kids.

I myself was shown a good nutritional example: My mother fed us whole foods (while not nearly 60–80 percent raw), very little sugar, and no white flour. She was a healthy weight and exercised regularly. She didn't talk to me about the whys of it all, but the example alone has had a powerful effect on my life, as you can see. That said, I completely rebelled while in her home and for some years afterward, in my 20s. The lack of junk food in my childhood diet, however, was not the reason for my rebellion. The power of addictive chemical properties in refined foods was. I fell for it, hard, in my 20s. I weighed more at 25 than I weigh now at 42. I had less energy, my skin was worse, and I had mood and sleep disturbances I no longer have, all because my diet indulged in sugar, white flour, meat, dairy, and so on.

So take a long-range view as you educate your children. Even if they stray now, that doesn't mean they won't embrace your way of life (healthy eating) later, when they achieve more maturity. The worst thing we can do is to educate them about nothing and figure that's for later—eat junk now, develop a taste for vegetables in adulthood because that's an "adult taste." *That philosophy has the highest probability of backfiring.*

And realize that Rome wasn't built in a day; education of your children can't be just one grand lecture. You have to talk to your kids on a regular basis about a variety of issues that will lead them toward the narrow path to good health in a world of crazy nutrition. As you read this book, or *12 Steps to Whole Foods*, or other nutrition books, consider as you read how you can adapt the information to share with your children.

5. Get your child's pint in: two sittings instead of one.

My kids sometimes come home from school and drink some of their green smoothie, and if I find that some still remains in the fridge, they finish it at dinner. Other families start with green smoothie for breakfast, which is a great idea. You don't have to push your children to finish it all at once. In fact, if it provides precursor live enzymes for two cooked meals or snacks, then all the better.

6. Require raw food (like green smoothie) before the child eats other things, being firm and consistent (never beg and plead).

This is what we do as adults, right? We eat our nutritious food before dessert. Otherwise, we get in trouble fast, with health and weight problems, since you can quickly eat far too many calorie-dense bites of food if that's what you start with. So it logically follows that we should teach our children the same.

Pediatricians often tell parents that they should "offer" good foods but not make a "big deal" about what small children eat. This sounds to me like weak counsel that will lead to junk-food addictions, because if you offer a bowl of steamed carrots and a plate of pizza, kids will take the pizza every time. (I watched this in action once, when 25 out of 25 children chose the pizza.) So would I, if I didn't know better. And a child doesn't know better.

My counsel is the virtual opposite of most pediatricians: Offer *only* healthy choices at home except on very rare occasions, if ever. That's where self-discipline and good decision-making is learned, in the home. Good choices are best learned when a child has a good example in a firm but kind *leader* in the home.

A parent who whines and begs a child to do anything—drinking the green smoothie being just one example—is a parent telling the child very distinctly, "I'm not in charge here." I have a friend who had a custom sign made for her home that says, "We do hard things here." I'm firm with my two children who sometimes resist, one of whom occasionally pitches a fit about drinking her green smoothie, and I just smile and say, "That's who we are in this family and that's what we do here." They can go play, or eat whatever else is offered, after the smoothie is gone. (If it helps you, you can borrow my moniker and be the Green Smoothie Girl. That certainly comes in handy at my house. I look at my daughter, cock my head to the side, and joke, "Come on now—you know I'm the Green Smoothie Girl. You really think anything is ever gonna change around here on this subject?")

Never beg or negotiate. The parent who begins to whine and cajole a resistant child has, in essence, put herself on the child's level. The immediate message to the child is that he or she is now in charge. Stay above the emotional drama and just persistently and pleasantly reiterate the nutritional standards in the home. Giving in and bringing back the junk food tells them Mom doesn't have self-discipline and can be manipulated easily.

My recalcitrant daughter is welcome to put a lid on her pint jar and put it back in the fridge. But when she gets hungry after school, she has to drink that before eating any popcorn or making herself some toast or a sandwich. If she hasn't finished it at dinnertime, it's at her place at the table. Again.

There's another purely common-sense reason to have children drink the green smoothie, or eat the green salad, first. And that's to provide enzymes to the stomach as the other food (cooked, without enzymes) arrive. This signals to the enzyme-manufacturing organs of the body such as the pancreas that you've got the digestive job covered. Then you aren't robbing metabolic processes of scarce enzymes to do digestive work. Always have your meals and snacks be 60–80 percent raw, and start with the raw food. This seems a daunting goal at first, but it's very achievable once the mindset is attained. I never eat cooked foods without eating raw foods first, and my children know this principle well, too.

7. Consider a reward system (only if your child is resistant and other efforts have failed).

I don't particularly love reward systems, but some parents have found this effective to avoid a war when it comes to food. It works particularly well with children who understand and respond to consequences (a very good sign, if they do, by the way, since we all navigate positive and negative consequences in life).

I would recommend that you don't use treats and junk food as reinforcements for good eating habits. That's confusing, even if many of us have that flawed logic in our own psyche. The idea that if we eat something good, we're now entitled to eat something bad is problematic and leads us to emotional eating problems.

Instead, think about what very specifically motivates your child, and make it something inexpensive for you, or something you really are willing to do. For many children, the very best reward is time spent with Mom and/or Dad. What about, for a month of drinking your green smoothie every day, you get a trip to the dollar store with Mom, or an ice skating excursion with Dad?

Remember to praise a child who is a "good eater." I often tell my older daughter that I'm impressed with her choices. I also link her good habits to the health benefits I see she has achieved, such as, "You have such beautiful skin. Most teenagers don't. You can thank your green smoothies for that!" Or, "Have you noticed that you're the only girl on your soccer team who never asks the coach to take her out? Why do you think that is?"

8. Make green smoothies into popsicles.

Especially in the summer, and especially for young children, this is a great way to pose a healthy habit as a treat. You can purchase inexpensive popsicle makers at Walmart or Target. You may want to make them a bit sweeter (with agave nectar or stevia) for this purpose, and you can add plain yogurt if you want to make them creamy. Add enough berries that the popsicles are not actually green. Don't even tell the kids what's in the popsicles!

9. Make green smoothies when kids aren't watching.

Kids who have never eaten much of anything nutritious (whom you plan to wean off the standard American diet) will be horrified watching you blend kale and celery for them to drink. Do it when they aren't there and don't tell them what's in it. I did a nutrition class recently for a group of young moms who brought their children with them. They all went off to play while I did the green smoothie demo. When I was done, we put the greens away and called the kids in. Every one of them slurped the smoothies up.

10. Add lots of berries or dark colors and put the smoothie in a pretty glass.

Green smoothies are so named because of their actual ingredients. There's no rule that they have to end up looking . . . well, green! Or yucky, for that matter. My favorite ingredient to make a smoothie purple (okay, sometimes more like brown, which is still better than green) is frozen mixed berries. At the time of this writing, they can be obtained most inexpensively at Costco (four pounds for $11), or seasonally in local buying groups to keep in your freezer. You can also add a beet to change the color of smoothies radically.

For slightly older children, pour your smoothies into a pretty or fun glass that is reserved for treats. Use fun straws. These ideas just make the experience a more positive one.

10

Ten Tips to Save Money as a GreenSmoothieGirl (or Guy)

After people get over the initial hurdle of wondering what a green smoothie tastes like, and finding out it can actually be quite nice, their next objection is the cost. "Those ingredients are expensive!" they say, or, "How much does a blender full of that stuff cost?!"

Overall, before offering my cost-saving tips, I want to point out that eating lots of raw greens can prevent so many health problems that you truly can't afford *not* to eat them. You'll surely save in the long run when you aren't dealing with the expensive side effects of illness, obesity, and the thousands of attendant risks of the typical American lifestyle.

That said, here are ten tips to save money—the first two will have an enormous cost-saving impact on your budget, if you're willing to invest a bit of cash and time up-front. The payoff of implementing just the top two ideas in this list can be very rewarding.

1. Learn to Garden

I cannot overstate the importance of learning to garden, which will make your greens virtually free throughout the spring, summer, and fall. And, with a little planning, you can have almost-free, organic green smoothie ingredients year-round. Grow a garden that features greens prominently. Learn to garden through the winter, and freeze the extra greens in the warm growing season.

Spinach, chard, and kale are very easy to grow in backyard or patio gardens, and at the end of the summer you can replant for a fall harvest that really explodes again in the spring right through the frost season. Chard, in particular, produces a massive amount of green food and does not bolt easily in hot weather; by staggering plantings, I harvest it from a few weeks after the spring frost until well after the last fall frost. Also consider that carrots, beets, turnips, radishes, and strawberries now offer a new food source for you, because the green parts of those plants you may have been throwing away before are perfect for your smoothies.

2. Invest in a Large Freezer

This is the second-highest-impact idea I can offer to those who are frugal or strapped for cash: Invest in a large freezer. Buy it used from Craigslist if necessary. I keep mine in the garage, and it's permanently packed with perishable items I buy in bulk like nuts and seeds, as well as gallon freezer bags containing the harvest from my garden that past summer/fall. Although I buy spinach through the winter and spring, I usually have enough chard, beet greens, and other green smoothie ingredients to get me through to the spring, when I have a new crop coming out of my garden.

3. Harvest Edible Weeds

A variety of greens can be harvested from empty lots in your neighborhood when the weather is warm. Edible weeds found in most climates include *lambsquarter leaves, nettles, morning glory,* and *purslane* (or even *thistle*). Purslane has a very mild flavor and texture for addition to smoothies; it's an unusually rich source of omega-3s and iron. Make sure you do not use weeds you are not certain are edible.

Dandelion weeds can sometimes be bitter but are plentiful in most climates, and I often throw a handful in the blender. Avoid picking these weeds in areas next to busy roadways, as greens absorb the toxins in car exhaust fumes. Also avoid any areas that have been sprayed with pesticides or weed killer. Dandelion greens are least bitter when they are picked in the spring before they bloom with yellow flowers.

4. Buy in Bulk

I highly recommend a membership at Costco. It usually carries huge (2.5 pounds) bags of washed spinach at lower prices than regular grocery and health food stores (only $3.99 where I live). That's 25–50 percent of what you'd spend on the 10-ounce bags of spinach for $1.99 to $3.99 at regular grocery stores. Bananas, pears, frozen strawberries, and frozen mixed berries are also much less expensive on a regular basis at Costco than in any grocery store where I live, except on the rare occasion those items are on sale elsewhere.

My brother and his wife once did a cost comparison of 20 items they buy regularly, and 19 of the 20 items were cheaper at Costco than the other grocery stores they shopped at. If you buy the membership, you must decide to shop there regularly, because if you do, you may get your entire membership fee back annually, based on usage. I get about $95 of my $100 back based on my family's buying habits. (Plus the membership is worth having for the cheapest gas in town.) See my video on GreenSmoothieGirl.com showing all the items I buy at Costco to save money and feed my family well.

5. Shop at Health Food Stores

Keep an eye on the contents of the health food stores in your area. At my local health food store, although organic bunches of kale, collards, and chard are admittedly more expensive than conventional produce, the bunches are much bigger, so the higher price is probably not higher per ounce. In this case, paying more is warranted for more reasons than just nutrition.

6. Freeze Fresh Fruit

Buy fruit on sale and in season, and freeze it before it goes bad. I have not thrown a single piece of fruit away in quite a few years, because if I see the bananas are getting black spots and I can't use them all, I peel them, break them into chunks, and put them in sandwich baggies in the freezer. I buy a lug or two of peaches when they're in season, and I wash and quarter them in baggies to freeze and last through the winter.

7. Freeze Fresh Greens

Greens, too, while they can't be frozen for salads and other purposes, can be easily frozen for later use in smoothies. No one will be able to tell. So you never have to let the spinach go bad again.

8. Buy Frozen Spinach

You can buy frozen spinach in the winter when fresh spinach is very expensive, and occasionally those boxes or bags of spinach in the freezer section are less expensive.

9. Support Local Growers

Find the community-supported agriculture and health-food-buying co-op groups in your area. They'll have great deals on organic produce that will bring your costs down.

10. Get to know the smaller markets in your area

I've found an Asian market near my home that has excellent prices on interesting greens like various cabbages (yu choy, bok choy, tatsoi, and quite a few others), as well as fresh ginger, a variety of vegetables, and young Thai coconuts.

11

Tips for Buying and Storing Greens and Fruit

Buying

Look for several things when you buy greens and fruit:

1. Do they look colorful and fresh? Avoid wilted produce or yellow or dry leaves.

2. Are they organic? They may cost more, but often at my own health food store, the organic bunches are larger than the conventional bunches at the regular grocery store, which is an important consideration. Know how much more you're willing to pay for organic items—25 percent more? 50 percent more? Base your decisions accordingly, but organic is worth more because nutrition is higher, according to many studies. A study published in *The Journal of Applied Nutrition* by Doctor's Data Lab in Illinois found that organic produce had higher

nutrient levels, twice the level in some cases, of conventional produce grown with pesticides.

Some greens are sponges for pesticides like DDT and other carcinogens, making organic purchases that much more important and worth your dollars. These high-accumulation greens include mustard greens, collard greens, and spinach.

3. Locally grown produce almost always tastes even better than the organic produce you can buy in the stores. That's because it's very fresh when you get it, not gassed and trucked across the country. Besides the fossil-fuel savings, you support local businesses and keep farmers from going out of business.

In addition to buying locally grown fruits and vegetables, I would also encourage you to ask your grocery store to stock local and organic produce. If enough people create the demand, the supply will follow.

Storing greens

Greens can be kept fresh for up to one week in the refrigerator, depending on how fresh they were when purchased. Twist off plastic bags that contain greens tightly or use a twist tie to keep out air and water and preserve their life.

Some ways to extend the life of your greens include the following:

1. Wash greens in advance of using them, and keep them in sealable Ziploc bags.

2. Put them in quart or half gallon jars, fill with water, and keep in the fridge (this idea contributed by a GreenSmoothie Girl.com reader).

3. When you realize that you won't be able to use all your greens before they go bad, chop them, put them in freezer

bags, and freeze them. Try to use them within a few weeks to minimize nutrient loss. I do use garden greens for six months, though, which isn't nutritionally ideal but gives me free produce year-round.

Make sure you wash your greens and fruit with a good veggie wash, which can be purchased at any health food store or online. I use Shaklee Basic H that I buy from someone local, and a gallon of concentrate, while expensive, lasts me a decade. I fill a spray bottle with water and add a tablespoon of the organic, biodegradable formula.

Some nutrients are lost through freezing, but it's still the best way to preserve foods. Dehydrating below 116 degrees is the second-best way to preserve nutrients.

After greens are blended, they begin to oxidize (cells begin to degenerate or "rust"). Ideally, we'd blend our drinks and consume them immediately. However, I'd encourage you to not feel guilty about keeping green smoothies in the refrigerator for up to 48 hours. If we're such purists that we insist on perfectly fresh smoothies, the end result for anyone living in the real world is that we just won't make green smoothies every day. And that would be the greater loss.

Sometimes practicality trumps the ideal situation. But screw a lid on your jar of smoothie tightly to minimize oxidation.

Selecting and storing fruit

Look for seasonal fruits in the summer that you enjoy in smoothies, and take them home by the lug or bushel. Wash, quarter, and pit them, put a handful for one smoothie recipe in a sandwich baggie, and freeze (or quick-freeze them on cookie sheets first so they don't clump together into a frozen mass). They can be used throughout the winter when pre-served this way.

Fruit often should be kept on the counter, rather than in the fridge, to ripen more naturally using the gases from ambient air. Fruit better kept out of the fridge include bananas, apples, peaches, and nectarines. Keep melons and other fruits in the fridge.

Here are additional tips:

Apples   Keep them on the counter, not in the fridge, so they don't become "mealy." They give off ethylene gas that ripens other fruit, so don't put them with potatoes (they'll grow sprouts) or other fruit you don't want to become overripe quickly. (On the other hand, if you want to speed up the ripening of bananas, put them in a brown paper bag with an apple.)

Avocados   Keep them on the counter or windowsill until they ripen. They're ripe when they become black and have a little "give" when you squeeze them slightly. Green avocados ripen nicely but can take two to seven days to do so. When they do become ripe, put them in the fridge to slow the ripening; this extends the time you have to use them by up to a week. When you use avocados, add a bit of fresh lemon juice to slow the oxidation that turns the flesh brown.

Bananas   Keep them on the counter or on a banana hook, not in the fridge where they're unable to ripen naturally. They'll overripen too quickly if a lot of them are together, so keep them separate as much as possible. Bananas are perfect to eat when they begin to develop a small number of dark spots and the green is gone; this is when the starches in the fruit have converted into sugars. When they begin to develop too many black spots, if you won't be using the bananas in the next day or two, simply peel them, break them into thirds, freeze in Ziploc sandwich bags, and use later in smoothies. If they're stuck together, just whack the bag of frozen banana chunks on the counter and they'll break apart. Or you can individually quick-freeze them on a cookie sheet before putting them in baggies. If you peel a banana from the bottom up, the little strings peel off better.

If you want to accelerate bananas' ripening, put them in a paper bag with an apple and roll the top closed. The apple's gases speed that process up so you won't have green bananas the next day.

Melons   Keep on the counter if ripening is needed, or in the fridge if they're ripe and you want to extend their life. You can tell a cantaloupe is ready to eat when you smell the indented end of it and it has a fragrant, ripe smell. When the cantaloupe is green, you can't smell anything. (This does not work with thin- and smooth-skinned melons like honeydew. The best test for a honeydew or watermelon is to buy one with rough, brownish "bug bites" on the skin.)

Oranges and other citrus   Keep in the fridge.

Pineapples and mangoes   Keep on the counter if ripening is needed, or in the fridge if they're ripe and you want to extend their life. You can tell a pineapple is ripe if it has yellow undertones rather than green under the brown scales, and you can easily pull one of the leaves out of the top. A ripe mango will have some "give" to it when squeezed slightly, and a green one will ripen on the counter or windowsill in one to five days.

Tomatoes   Keep them on the counter rather than in the fridge to avoid them becoming "mealy," which is an unpleasant texture for most recipes.

12

Grow Your Own Greens

Why garden?

Planting a garden is the best way to make green smoothies inexpensive. It also enables you to have control over the quality of your food, as you can garden organically very easily. It has two other side benefits: self-reliance in an emergency and helping you teach your children good work and reward principles.

People who garden tend to eat much more fresh produce and have an advantage in any kind of emergency situation, such as job loss. It's an excellent habit to cultivate, to teach children the "law of the harvest" very directly, that what you sow (and make an effort at), you reap.

Saundra Lorenz and fellow researchers at Texas A&M University discovered that when children spent 30 minutes weekly gardening, they were more likely to eat vegetables. Lorenz pointed out that young children often think food comes from a grocery store, and letting them work in a garden helps them make a connection to their food source, making whole plant foods more appealing.

My children tend the garden and pick weeds throughout the summer; they get very excited about bringing food in for our table later in the summer. We plant radishes, not because I particularly like them, but because they're the "short-term reinforcer" for the new little gardener: only a few weeks after planting the seeds, they're ready for small children with short attention spans to pick. Being able to use the radish tops in smoothies teaches them the principle of "reduce, reuse, recycle" that they now hear in school but often don't see practiced in American homes.

Many gardeners love to grow vegetables and then wonder what to do with it all when the plants offer up a yield. That's the beauty of your new green smoothie habit: a place to use all kinds of crazy green food, every day. And what you can't use, you can freeze.

My religion endorses a set of modern scripture (revealed in the 1830s) called The Doctrine and Covenants, and I quote Section 89, verses 10 and 11 following. People of the LDS (Mormon) faith believe that God is speaking directly to the people of our day about our diet: "Verily I say unto you, all wholesome herbs God hath ordained for the constitution, nature, and use of man—Every herb in the season thereof, and every fruit in the season thereof; all these to be used with prudence and thanksgiving."

What does this mean, to use herbs and fruits in the season thereof? Some theorize that our food supply is designed to provide the nutrients we need, precisely in the time of year that we need them. Some experts and ancient Eastern philosophies think that certain vitamins and minerals are important for the functions performed by the body in various parts of the year—that some times are for cleansing, some are for building, some are for working, etc.

This would fit well with any theory about God providing for his children's needs, or any theory about a world evolving to meet the needs of its inhabitants. And, of course, that suggests that the very best foods for us are the ones provided in our own soil, in the season those seeds were meant to grow. In other words, for instance, spinach and strawberries are needed by the body in the spring and fall, and cabbage in the late fall.

Another advantage to growing your own food is your reduced dependence on fossil fuels. Our food supply has become very pricey in terms of fossil fuels utilized to put our food on boats, trucks, and airplanes. We have access to produce from all over the globe, but at what cost? When we buy local produce or, even better, grow our own, our carbon footprint becomes much smaller and we contribute to making the world a better place for those who will come after us.

Having your hands and feet in contact with the earth is energizing in a very elemental way. We were meant to have contact with the ground and, in fact, we pick up massive antioxidants from "grounding"—our feet being in contact with earth. We were meant to be in the sun, as well. Exposure to sun gives us much-needed vitamin D that must be obtained to work with calcium to build bone mass. Sunshine also gives us a sense of peaceful well-being and connection to life and nature.

What you'll need

You'll need a garden space (ideally with wood square-foot boxes) or pots for gardening on a patio if you have no backyard (and a trellis if you want to plant vining vegetables).

You may wish to buy compost to add to the soil, and consider building one or more compost boxes in your backyard to reuse plant waste. Composted materials should be partly green (your food scraps) and partly brown (dead leaves, for instance), and should be turned several times over the course of several months as they decompose. Any compost pile should take a few months to one year to break down into a rich fertilizer for use in your garden.

You'll need a package of non-hybridized, chemically untreated seeds for each of the vegetables you'd like to grow. These are called "heirloom" seeds, and a good source is www.heirloomseeds.com. Or, on May 1 in most climates, you may purchase seedlings for tomatoes, peppers, cabbage, and many other plants from your local nursery.

Consider purchasing a new or used full-sized freezer to put in the garage. After gardening, this is the second-best way to save money eating a plant-based diet. It can dramatically extend the life of your garden produce, giving you vegetables and fruits through the winter. It also allows you to buy seeds and nuts in bulk through co-ops.

What if I have no space?

Many communities offer gardening space for free or for a very small fee, so ask your city about its resources. When I was a young, married college student living in apartments, we still had huge gardens. That's because one year we asked an elderly neighbor with unused garden space to let us use it, and another year we used the university community garden plots. "Where there's a will there's a way" comes to mind. Several years ago, with a newly built house and no landscaping in yet, I told my church congregation that we were without a garden and if anyone had extra produce, to let me know. We've never eaten so well as we did that summer!

You can also use pots on the smallest of patios or porches. I know people who have an abundant harvest by vining plants up their trellises and making ingenious use of pots. A small four-by-four-foot homemade grow box can also sit on concrete, and the six inches of dirt in it is enough to grow most crops. I once participated in a reality TV show where, to improve the family's fast-food-only nutrition, I directed the TV crew to build an impressive six-by-six-foot-square gardening grow box on the family's concrete skateboarding half-pipe in the tiny backyard! I knew they loved salsa, so it contained tomatoes, peppers, onions, cilantro, and even some flowers.

What should I grow?

Here are greens and fruits you can grow (and some root vegetables that have greens you can use), depending on the space you have. Some (like zucchini) aren't what you traditionally think of as greens, but you can certainly hide some in your smoothies.

Beets	Cabbage	Carrots
Endive	Escarole	Goji berries
Kale	Lettuce (all varieties)	Mesclun (mixed greens)
Radishes	Raspberries	Spinach
Strawberries (perennials)	Swiss chard	Zucchini

How do I grow greens?

Greens do best in a good loam or heavier soil, rather than

light, sandy soils. They do well when manure is added to the soil in the fall and given time over the winter to become part of the soil. Chicken manure, which has the highest nitrogen levels, is the best because leafy greens use nitrogen heavily. Don't add "green" (or fresh) manure in the spring right before planting. If you do fertilize in the spring, make sure to use aged material that will not "burn" your fledgling plants. (I have learned this lesson the hard way.)

Manure provides constant levels of nutrients for the plant, perfect for organic gardening. Giving your plants chemical fertilizers is the equivalent of you or me taking a synthetic vitamin: It's a shock of less-helpful nutrients, followed by starvation until the next fertilization.

Because you'll want a steady stream of greens for your smoothies over the course of many months, stagger your plantings. Usually if you have an invasion of pests, they'll focus on one patch and leave earlier plantings alone. This gives you time to deal with the pests before they overrun more of your garden.

Keep in mind that tender greens such as lettuce and arugula need to be harvested when they're young. Otherwise they get bitter. Staggered plantings are even more important if you want to extend your yield.

In general, greens need about an inch of water per week. Especially in the hottest part of the summer, spread that over two waterings per week. After the seed sprouts and you see a green shoot above ground, keeping the soil constantly moist is no longer necessary.

Pick your greens in the morning or evening, not in the heat of the day. They'll taste better and last longer in the fridge.

What about organic produce?

Besides cost savings and dramatically improved taste, home-grown vegetables have another huge advantage: They're easily grown organically. Some studies show that organic produce has higher concentrations of vitamins and minerals, and other studies have found that "conventional" (sprayed) produce is nutritionally equal to organic. The jury is out on whether nutrient levels are higher, but what is crystal clear is that non-sprayed produce is lower in toxic pesticide and herbicide residue. If you cannot afford organic produce (and even if you can), growing greens in your garden is an excellent option. If you do purchase conventional greens, using a quality vegetable wash (available at health food stores or online) and rinsing well will help reduce pesticide residues significantly. Remember that animal protein has higher concentrations of the same toxins because they build up in the organs and flesh, so don't make a decision to stay away from produce if conventional is the only kind you have access to. Alternative foods are worse.

I like to support local growers rather than international conglomerates wherever possible. Shipping food all over the planet is unique to the generations currently living on Earth. This practice consumes a lot of nonrenewable energy. One of the best things about gardening is a smaller carbon footprint, leaving more resources for future generations.

Why should I consider square-foot gardening?

For limited spaces, or to make the most of the space you have, I highly recommend square-foot gardening, which maximizes the yield per foot of space. You're gardening based on squares instead of rows, which lets you get twice the amount of produce out of half the space.

In one square foot, you might have nine beets, or four lettuce heads, or one corn stalk or tomato plant. This method is eco-friendly because you use much less water than with traditional gardening. You also have less weeding and a space designed for better access, since the grow boxes are up off the ground. The author of the system says that square-foot gardening uses 80 percent less space, time (especially weeding), water, and money than the traditional method.

I also recommend that you plan ahead to stagger plantings (planting hardier greens and vegetables as early as possible) so that your harvest doesn't come all at once, providing much more than you need. With staggered plantings, you enjoy vegetables for an extended period of time. Square-foot gardening is the perfect way to achieve that: I go out every Saturday from April onward, planting just a few squares each week of greens, beets, corn, and some other crops that I like to extend.

If you live in climates that are cold and snowy through the winter, you can plant a few crops as early as three to five weeks before the last spring frost, as indicated below. In Utah, we plan on that being May 1, though on a rare occasion it is later—if you're new to gardening, you'll have to get used to the fact that you have no guarantees in nature! Warm-weather crops are planted on May 1 (and then hold your breath and cover your tomatoes if the forecast calls for a freeze). But here are a few exceptions:

You can plant as early as the *first week in April*:

Peas and spinach from seed; broccoli and cabbage from seedlings.

You can plant as early as the *second week in April*:

Beets, carrots, radishes, lettuce, and chard from seeds; onion sets.

Be sure to build boxes with untreated lumber that will not leach chemicals into your soil and, therefore, your food. Boxes sit on top of the ground and can be 4' x 4', 4' x 6', or even 2' x 2'. You can use string tied around nails or screws to divide the boxes into squares that are 1' x 1'.

I plan my square-foot garden by drawing tables that match each of my boxes, like this 6' x 4' box below. I plan for staggered plantings by detailing the date I want to plant that crop in each box. Then I mark each square after I plant it with a check mark to keep track of what to water.

Carrots Apr. 1	Spinach Apr. 1	Spinach Apr. 8	Spinach Apr. 15	Chard Apr. 1	Chard Apr. 8
Carrots Apr. 8	Spinach Apr. 1	Spinach Apr. 8	Spinach Apr. 15	Radishes May 1	Radishes May 1
Carrots Apr. 15	Spinach Apr. 1	Spinach Apr. 8	Spinach Apr. 15	Beets May 1	Radishes April 15
Carrots Apr. 22	Spinach Apr. 1	Spinach Apr. 8	Spinach Apr. 15	Beets May 15	Radishes May 1

Plant 16 per square: radishes, carrots
Plant 9 per square: beets, spinach
Plant 4 per square: lettuce, chard, parsley
Plant 1 per square: cabbage, kale

Water newly planted crops every day until you see the plant above ground. (If the seed dries out, it dies.) After the plant appears, you can water it every three days (or two if it's very hot outside during the day).

One of the best reasons to do square-foot gardening is that you can often get two crops out of one square in one season. For instance, in April, you can plant cool-weather-loving lettuce, which matures quickly. Then you can pick it around the end of May, add some compost to that square, and plant some radishes or beets in that square.

For detailed information on this method of gardening, I recommend *Square Foot Gardening* by Mel Bartholomew. You can learn more about vining in the square-foot method, building trellises for vines (I use the fence next to my garden, but we did build metal trellises at our last home), how to plant quick-to-grow small vegetables such as radishes in the same square around a plant like bell pepper that takes some time to mature, and much more.

How do I keep the pests away without using chemicals?

Lots of natural and safe techniques can help the good organisms in your garden thrive while killing the bad ones.

Employ companion planting   Plant a square of marigolds, onions, or garlic interspersed throughout your gardening boxes, because pests tend to avoid these plants.

Use garlic, onions, hot peppers   They kill soft-body insects and paralyze flying insects, as well as serving as a fungicide and repelling rabbits. Liquefy some of these vegetables in water in your high-power blender and spray the mixture on plants and soil. (Pour boiling water mixed with garlic on ant mounds.)

Use apple cider vinegar, ground cloves   Use 1–2 tablespoons per gallon of water for a mild fungicide or acidic liquid fertilizer that also contains many trace elements as a fertilizer. Cloves kill flying insects.

Use cornmeal, diatomaceous earth   Sprinkle on the ground or work into the top inch of soil. Diatomaceous earth can work in your soil for many years; it's the petrified remains of insects and shreds the digestive system of bugs and dehydrates them. (It will kill bees, so avoid spraying it, as we have a honeybee shortage.)

Set traps   Around a can or cut-off milk jug containing rotten fruit, pour a liquid made of water with 2 tablespoons each of dish soap and vegetable oil to kill pests, and, optionally, 2 tablespoons of molasses to attract more pests.

Kill snails and slugs   Sprinkle calcium carbonate products like lime, dolomite, or crushed eggshells on soil where snails and slugs live; antifungal properties are another advantage.

Use acidic water   You can also spray the leaves of your plants with acid water if you have a water ionizer (a topic covered on GreenSmoothieGirl.com in *12 Steps to Whole Foods*) to kill many pests.

Plant vines later   According to old-timer gardeners, cucumbers and squash do better when planted June 1. Often when I jump the gun and plant on May 1, they end up dead of pest problems. When I wait, they grow and bloom quickly and produce well.

Feel free to mix and match, to make teas of a variety of the natural pest-repelling compounds listed above.

How can I get green produce in the winter?

If you want to extend the life of your garden and grow cold-weather greens without an expensive and complicated greenhouse, I highly recommend *Four-Season Harvest: Organic Vegetables from Your Home Garden All Year Long* by Eliot Coleman. The author lives in Maine and gets hardy greens like mache and spinach throughout the winter, using modifications to the square-foot gardening boxes that protect plants and allow the sun to warm them through plexiglass. You can also interact with others and ask questions about the four-season harvest online, where support communities are thriving.

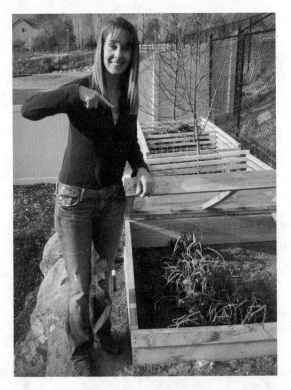

The photo above is of me opening one of my winter grow boxes in March 2008, after an entire (bitterly cold) winter of complete neglect on my part. I had planted onion, spinach, and chard in the late fall, and, to my delight, I found them green and growing at the end of March.

How do I compost?

As someone who eats a lot of plant food, you have many peels and other vegetable waste that should be going to good use, providing recycled nutrition to your plants (and later, you). We have three compost piles that we rotate to make good soil supplementation for our garden. We throw vegetable waste and grass clippings into the first one until we have enough, and then we mix that "green" layer with the "brown" layer of leaves or sawdust. When our neighbors are bagging their leaves in the fall, we take some home, poke holes in the bags, and let the water from rain and snow percolate through the bags to decompose their contents, in addition to using our own (unbagged) leaves to mix with "green" compost.

After we stop adding to one compost pile, we throw our clippings and peels into the second pile, while the first one is decomposing for use in the next planting. By rotating the three piles, we have one that is ready to use in gardening, one

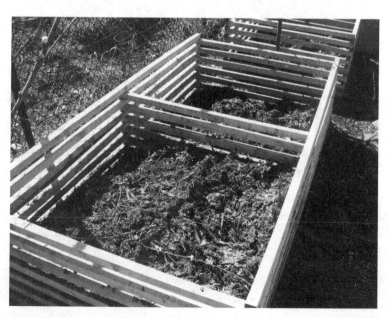

we are actively adding to, and a third that we're not adding to, but still needs some decomposition time.

Our compost piles also create some bizarre benefits and drama unrelated to "green" recycling and good nutrition. Our dogs immediately eat some of the produce peels, melon guts, and other waste that we throw in the boxes, which tells me that they want better nutrition than typical dog food made of animal products provides. Also, during the winter of 2007/08, a family of ferrets took up residence in one of our boxes, and a family of quail in another box!

Which are the easiest green smoothie ingredients to grow?

My favorite green to grow is chard, because it's easy to grow and very prolific—it continues to produce long after spinach has gone to seed. I have fresh chard from May through October, literally half the year, despite being in a cold climate. You can cut stalks of chard off the plant, and it just regrows! Freezing my abundant chard harvest gets me through the winter making green smoothies, too, so I can access this food virtually year-round. I buy rainbow-colored and regular Swiss chard seeds for variety in nutrition.

I do love spinach, and I recommend planting it as early as possible in the spring, and planting at the beginning of the fall as well—it will be dormant through the winter and suddenly explode with growth in the very early spring, giving you a harvest long before you could've planted and cultivated it. If you have hot summers, you won't have spinach after the temperature hits about 90 degrees, because it does "bolt" (go to seed) quite easily.

I also find beets very easy to grow and multi-purpose in that I love both the below-ground vegetable and the green, for very different recipes. I thin the beet greens by cutting a few stalks every time I go out to the garden for spinach and chard. The beets take a few months to grow, but feel free to use some of the beet greens early (just leave some of them to aid the growth of the root vegetable).

To summarize, grow these staple ingredients for six months of fresh greens and six months of frozen greens, more or less depending on your climate and growing season:

- Beets
- Chard
- Lettuces
- Radishes
- Turnips
- Cabbage
- Kale
- Mache
- Spinach

13

The Green Smoothies Diet

The three plans in this chapter are designed to help you get the most out of your green smoothies. Whether you want to quickly rid your body of toxins, lose weight in a safe and healthy way, or completely change the way you live and become a GreenSmoothieGirl or Guy, here you'll find the plan that will help you do it in a safe and healthy way.

Three-Day Green Fast (Detox)

For those transitioning from a fairly standard American diet, I recommend using this program only after a few weeks or even months of drinking a quart of green smoothie daily. The detoxification that can sometimes result from a green-smoothie cleanse, if your body is highly toxic, can be a shock to the body's systems. How do you know if you're highly toxic? Lots of chronic health conditions are just one sign. Another is a lifetime of drinking alcohol or smoking; a long period of time eating processed foods, soft drinks, and meat and dairy; and/or a habit of not drinking enough water.

So working your way up to a cleanse program like this, with slower cleansing by having a quart of green smoothie daily, is a good idea. You can skip this preliminary step if you've been eating lots of whole foods and raw vegetables and fruit for two months or more. Read "What To Do about a Cleansing Reaction" (page 111) in this book for a primer on what to expect as your body begins to use the excellent raw materials you provide to clean house and to repair and rebuild many damaged or diseased organs and functions in your body.

This three-day detox is easy, and great for:

- Losing several pounds quickly
- Giving the kidneys, liver, and digestive system a much-needed rest, reducing risk for kidney and gallstones or breaking up existing stones
- Recovering from a long trip or a period of poor eating
- Clearing impurities through your skin and achieving better skin health

You can undertake this detoxification program while living your normal life, with all its demands. You should be able to go to work, play your sports or work out like you normally do, and/or look after children. The beauty of it, rather than complete fasting, is that you'll have blood sugar support, good nutrition, and enough calories to maintain energy.

You may choose any of the recipes in this book to use in your three days. Stock up on the ingredients you'll need in advance. Make your full day of green smoothies early in the morning (about 96 ounces) so that they're prepared and waiting for you any time you're hungry, making the temptation to eat other things less intense.

WHAT TO EAT:

Eat nothing but green smoothies and, in between, drink 8–10 glasses of pure (preferably alkaline) water.

Drink as much green smoothie as you want (any one of the recipes in this book that makes 3 quarts is a good one-day supply).

Add 1–2 tablespoons of flax oil, or an avocado, to your pitcher of green smoothie daily.

You may get hungry occasionally, but have some green smoothie whenever you want food.

Thirty-Day Fat Burner Cleanse (Weight loss)

This more significant program involves a commitment of a greater period of time, with greater gains, including:

- Losing ten pounds or more (for those needing to lose weight)
- Significantly strengthening organs of elimination
- Breaking up and eliminating much of the years' worth of hardened mucoid plaque in the 100-plus feet of the digestive tract
- Regaining colonic regularity with soft but formed stool
- Beginning to reverse some health conditions, especially with a transition to the "Green Smoothie for Life" program when you're done

This program involves drinking half a gallon of green smoothies daily, plus eating other raw plant foods only. If you crave cooked food, steam some vegetables or bake a potato. Eat freely of these foods (many appropriate recipes are found in *12 Steps to Whole Foods* at GreenSmoothieGirl.com):

Green salads and other raw salads

Sprouted grains, legumes, nuts, and seeds

Fruits (such as berries, bananas, citrus such as oranges and grapefruit, tropical fruits such as mangoes and pineapples, cherries, apples, pears)

Vegetables of all kinds, such as yams or sweet potatoes, green beans, carrots, cauliflower, broccoli, asparagus, beets, turnips, celery, artichokes

Fresh or dried herbs such as basil, mint, oregano, tarragon

Up to ¼ cup seeds like flax, chia, sunflower, sesame, pumpkin, especially sprouted (soaked overnight)

Up to ¼ cup nuts like raw almonds, cashews, filberts, macadamias (not salted/roasted varieties)

Optionally, you may eat:

Small amounts of raw sauces and dressings, cold-pressed oils, or desserts made from raw ingredients

Crackers made from seeds, nuts, and vegetables with a dehydrator

Avoid these foods:

Coffee, tea, and alcohol

White flour

Refined sugars and chemical sweeteners (corn syrup, white sugar, NutraSweet, Splenda, etc.)

Beef, poultry, fish, shellfish, pork

Dairy products

Oils except small amounts of virgin, cold-processed oils (like olive or coconut)

Green Smoothie for Life
(Permanent lifestyle change)

Drinking a quart of green smoothie daily, for life, according to GreenSmoothieGirl.com research, achieves:

- Ideal weight for the long term
- Significantly reduced risk of disease
- Dramatic increase in energy
- A permanent change in digestive patterns, eliminating within 12–24 hours of eating
- Decreased desire for refined sugar
- Over the first year, elimination of heavy buildup of mucoid plaque in the digestive system as well as heavy metals and other toxic materials
- Reversal of mineral deficiency issues, so that nails strengthen and grow faster, hair thickens, and gray hair possibly returns to its natural color
- Increased sex drive and mitigated PMS symptoms or menstrual irregularity

This program, Green Smoothie for Life, is the lifestyle that this book, my efforts as a book author and lecturer, and my example intend to promote. It's the program that my family and I have followed for many years with great success, even while traveling, going to parties, and eating in restaurants as we all do, living in the "real world." That is, making a commitment to drinking a quart of green smoothie every day, and eating a "high raw" diet. Even if you want to live in the "real world" where eating 100 percent raw plant food is difficult, nigh unto impossible, virtually anyone can commit to eating 60–80 percent raw every day.

This, then, is a program for excellent health, high energy, minimal disease risk, and ideal weight. Do this every day:

- Drink 1 quart or more of green smoothie daily (any time—breakfast, lunch, snack—in two or more sittings, whenever you want)
- Eat 60–80 percent raw plant food including greens, vegetables, fruits, nuts, seeds, and sprouted grains/legumes/nuts/seeds
- Eat the remainder of the diet with mostly whole grains and legumes, or steamed or lightly sautéed vegetables
- Eat less than 5 percent animal protein (preferably none except for yogurt or kefir daily)
- Eliminate or rarely eat sugar, white flour, animal flesh and dairy, refined salt, fast foods, and any other processed foods

On my website and blogs, I often sing the praises of a colon-cleanse regimen called Arise & Shine (ariseandshine. com). The good news is that, while this somewhat expensive and time-consuming cleanse achieves phenomenal results in just 28 days or less, it isn't the only way to clean out years' worth of garbage accumulated in your 100-plus feet of digestive tract.

If you adhere to the program above and minimize or completely eliminate meat and processed foods, you'll, over time, achieve very impressive cleansing, including breaking up and eliminating hardened mucoid plaque that Dr. Bernard Jensen documented extensively in his studies of thousands of cleanse patients. You can trust green blended foods to do their work of dragging the digestive system and absorbing toxins, even those that have been there for decades. It will take longer than three to four weeks on the Arise & Shine cleanse, but it's highly effective over a longer period of time if you commit and make a lifestyle change.

What to Do about a Cleansing Reaction

Perhaps the most confusing thing about undertaking a committed green smoothie habit is when you're expecting good results and instead you feel pretty terrible. This is a common consequence, unfortunately, yet only a short-term one. When the body begins to recognize new, good materials coming in, all its systems grab the opportunity to begin using those materials to clean house and begin rebuilding. Many organs of elimination, including the colon, liver, kidneys, skin, and lymph system, go into high gear. They can sometimes be overwhelmed and clogged by a deluge of toxins trying to "get out" through various avenues.

Over 80 percent of the respondents in my research reported no cleansing reactions at all as they began their new habit of drinking at least a pint of green smoothie at least three times a week. (And cleansing reactions can be delayed, as well—they don't always take place immediately as you begin a new health habit.) However, a minority of people do experience one or more symptoms. These reactions were reported by at least one person in my study, with the first several answers being reported by several people and the last half of the list reported by only one person:

- Headaches
- Diarrhea
- Bloating
- Cramps
- Vertigo
- Fainting
- Runny nose
- Skin breakouts
- Nausea
- Intestinal gas
- Constipation
- Dizziness
- Lethargy or weakness
- Mucus in the back of the throat

- Liver pain
- Depression

- Mood swings
- Emotional crisis

What should you do, then, if you experience any of these symptoms? For starters, recognize symptoms of discomfort as what they are: a good thing—and don't abandon a great new habit, though you may wish to slow down by decreasing your smoothie consumption for a few days.

Second, drink extra water to flush out built-up toxins that need help evacuating. That should be about eight glasses of water for the average person, perhaps more for people who have larger builds. Drink water 20 minutes or more before a meal, or two hours or more after a meal, so the water does not dilute gastric juices when food is in the stomach. Tips for getting enough water into your schedule include, first, getting in the habit of drinking a pint immediately upon waking up, because you wake up dehydrated. Second, drink a glass of water every time you pass a drinking fountain during your workday. (You don't have to drink it from the water fountain if you bring higher-quality water, but that can be your reminder.) Third, drink a glass or two when you're preparing dinner (since dinner prep usually takes 20 minutes or more). Finally, get in the habit of always taking a water bottle with you in the car, to and from work or the gym or running errands.

Some believe that the "cleansing reaction" is just a cop-out by those in "alternative health" fields when we don't know what a health problem is. However, if you begin to undertake good nutrition, or work with others who do, you cannot help but notice how common this phenomenon is. The frequency of "cleansing reactions" reported by green smoothie drinkers in my research also is evidence of this. We may chalk up far too much to this phenomenon, but, on the other hand, the body is constantly cleaning house, and with the buildup of a variety of chemicals and digestive-tract sludges from the modern diet in various organs of the body, it's truly no wonder that we feel ill when too much elimination takes place at once.

When I was 25, I was in the middle of a period of having left behind the solid nutritional education and background I'd come from. I was at work one winter day, and I was totally sick. I was 15 pounds overweight, lacking energy every day, and discouraged that I had been unable to conceive for several years. But that particular day I was downright ill with some kind of virus. I told my boss I was going home, but on the way home I stopped at Dr. Christopher's Herb Shoppe in Orem, Utah. I went in and bought a Champion Juicer to get started on my new health kick.

Interestingly, the employee there, Carolyn, was doing a demo of the juicer at that moment. (That was my first time in that store, but 15 years later, I believe she still works there!) She was telling everyone how she and her husband had measured their poop! They scooped it out of the toilet, placed it on newspaper end to end, and measured it to see if it was 18 inches long like it should be. She said, "You should be eliminating from here to here, every day!" (She held up her arm and pointed to the length from her elbow to the tips of her fingers.)

My jaw was on the floor. I was horrified. "I am so outta here," I thought. (Some of you are thinking the same thing, reading this. Stay with me.) I couldn't wait to see my husband that night and mock the wacko at the health food store. (For years, he brought it up and made jokes, long after I became a big believer in the very principles Carolyn was teaching that day and quit mocking them.) I did, despite my incredulity, stop to buy the juicer as I bolted for the door, muttering under my breath.

My, how things have changed! Not that I am as earnestly open with the subject of elimination as Carolyn was. But, even if talking about elimination is new for you now, someday you might feel quite differently about it. (If you doubt me, just sit a while with elderly people, who are generally preoccupied with the topic.) Carolyn planted a seed, which actually helped me a lot, even if it was a few years later when I began to learn and embrace what she already knew and I couldn't handle at the time.

What about laxatives?

It's critically important that we keep the colon and lower intestine clean and powerfully peristaltic (that is, contracting and moving naturally). The answer isn't to gag down some chemically reduced Metamucil stirred into water while eating the Atkins Diet, like so many Americans are doing. When I discuss this with Atkins followers, mentioning the importance of plant fiber, they say, "Oh, I'm covered. I chug Metamucil (or FiberCon) like crazy."

Dr. Jensen says 95 percent of the millions of dollars spent annually on laxatives are only stimulating the bowel by irritating and harming it. If you want to use a very effective natural laxative that will stimulate without causing diarrhea or irritating the colon, have the herb Cascara Sagrada on hand. (But the best thing to prevent constipation in the first place, of course, is a daily green smoothie habit.)

Laxatives do one or more of three things. They (1) increase the amount of liquid retained in the feces, (2) act as a lubricant, or (3) irritate, poison, and/or chemically stimulate muscle walls to cause abnormal contractions. If you have diarrhea, it's due to one or more of these four reasons: (1) excessive use of laxatives, (2) stress, (3) infection in the GI tract/

colon, or (4) toxins in the bowel. These chemicals are absorbed through lymph and blood vessels and end up in various parts of the body. They damage the normal ability of the bowel to eliminate on its own, tiring out muscles by keeping them constantly stimulated.

Your blood recirculates through the colon, and toxicity in that part of your body is then spread to other parts of the body. Doctors will tell you this isn't so. But Dr. Jensen (who originally believed that) noticed that when a person retained water in the colon from enemas, he eliminated a lot of urine afterward. If the water in the colon is being taken back up to the kidneys, how, then, are none of the impurities in the colon being recirculated? In his urinalyses, Dr. Jensen used to test for *indican* level (toxic material taken back to the kidneys from the colon), though modern doctors don't.

By studying thousands of colons and eliminations, Jensen showed that the bowel is key to our health. Perhaps the most valuable thing I learned as a young mother is to give my children a simple enema with a syringe when they got a fever. I never met a fever that didn't reduce immediately after eliminating blockage in a little person's body.

The way to heal the bowel is through diet that promotes excellent nerve and muscle tone, with clean, pink, highly peristaltic tissues. And what's that diet? Lots of clean water, and lots of bulky greens, vegetables, fruits, legumes, whole grains, nuts, and seeds. The GreenSmoothieGirl diet prevents ulcerations, diverticulitis, spastic bowel, IBS, strictures, adhesions, colitis, and gas/flatulence that are affecting increasing numbers of people in the Western world.

Additionally, you can do a very simple thing to get off laxatives and become more regular. Wake up your digestive system every morning as you wake up, before you get out of bed.

Massage your ascending, transverse, and descending colon with your hands or a tennis ball. Massage deeply, starting in the lower right of your pelvis, work straight upwards, then massage right to left across your belly button, and straight down on the left. Then get up and start your day with two glasses of water. Sometime every day, drink a full quart of green smoothie. These are very effective natural laxatives that have the potential to end your digestive problems forever and virtually eliminate your risk of hemorrhoids, colon cancer, diverticulitis, Crohn's disease, Irritable Bowel Syndrome, and so many other miserable ailments afflicting those living in the wake of destruction created by processed food.

The importance of colon cleansing

Dr. Bernard Jensen is basically the poo guru of all time (for more about *Dr. Jensen's Guide to Better Bowel Care: A Complete Program for Tissue Cleansing through Bowel Management* and other books, see the book reviews on GreenSmoothieGirl. com). Dr. Jensen worked with 10,000 patients and documented his scientific findings on intestinal health and cleansing through thousands of photos. His photos will put to rest any scoffing your doctor may do at the need for, or results of, colon cleansing. Then you can do your own experiments so that you're not straining credulity to believe that you do, in fact, have hardened mucoid plaque in your body that shouldn't be there and can be eliminated.

You always hear about how when Elvis Presley and John Wayne were autopsied, they had 10 or 20 pounds of impacted fecal material in their digestive tracts due to chronic constipation. I have no idea if that's urban legend, but Dr. Jensen proved that this is the case in most, if not all, of us.

Does your doctor scoff at the idea of cleansing, at the idea that there's a buildup of hardened mucoid plaque in the digestive tract from eating meat and processed food and chemicals? Or, if you look around online, you can find a doctor or two saying this doesn't happen. That's astonishing to me. Having experienced its elimination for myself, this is not something I have to take on faith after purely academic study, and you can see for yourself. Look at the inside of many people's colons, both diseased and healthy, on Dr. Shinya's video clip found on YouTube (search for "Dr. Shinya Kangen water").

Dr. Bernard Jensen worked on tens of thousands of human colons. He once measured three gallons of hard, toxic material eliminated from one person in one cleansing treatment. You eliminate every day, you say? Your doctor and the medical textbooks (including pediatrics') say that one bowel movement every five days is fine and normal? Jensen says he knew a woman who eliminated five times a day but when he autopsied her after her death, the opening through her colon was the diameter of a pencil, even though the diameter of the vessel itself was nine inches.

It's not what's coming out that's a problem. It's what's staying in.

If you undertake a colon cleanse and go to a professional for colonics at the end of it, you may also evacuate fairly large intestinal parasites. Fortunately, through cleansing and clean eating, I have been parasite-free for years. When my blood is tested, it's not perfect, but it doesn't contain any parasites, and I'm told that is very rare. (Avoiding meat is key in this.) When all putrefaction is removed from the body and we eat a plant-based, whole-foods diet, we are no longer breeding grounds for bacteria, fungus, molds, viruses, and their dangerous byproducts, mycotoxins.

Sir Arbuthnut Lane was a surgeon for the King of England and specialized in bowel issues. He removed parts of the colon and sewed the rest back together, and in the course of his practice, he noticed that many times, patients after surgery would have goiters or arthritis disappear, or see other dramatic health improvements. Often, seemingly unrelated maladies improved after removing diseased sections of the colon.

He became so aware of how toxic digestive systems are linked to the other organs of the body that he spent the last 25 years of his life teaching people nutrition, rather than performing surgery. He said this:

> All maladies are due to the lack of certain food principles, such as mineral salts or vitamins, to the absence of the normal defenses of the body, such as the natural protective flora. When this occurs, toxic bacteria invade the lower alimentary canal, and the poisons thus generated pollute the bloodstream and gradually deteriorate and destroy every tissue, gland and organ of the body.

If pictures speak a thousand words, look at the color photos in Bernard Jensen's book. (You can also find this kind of thing by googling on the Internet.) They show rubbery material expelled from many colons during colemas (home colonics) and a cleansing program. Often, pieces are several feet long, the precise shape of specific parts of the bowel. These can be as hard as tire rubber, held up with tongs. Perhaps any modern doctor who insists this doesn't happen in the human digestive tract has spent too much time prescribing drugs and not enough time actually studying the inside of that organ. Hardened plaque like that is not simply the elimination of the capsules of loose herbs and bentonite clay used in the cleanse program.

When Dr. Jensen attended National College in Chicago, they performed surgeries on 300 people. Their histories said that 285 claimed they weren't constipated, and 15 claimed they were. Autopsies showed the exact opposite: 285 were constipated (despite reports that they had up to 5–6 bowel movements a day), and in some of them, "the bowel walls were encrusted with material (in one case peanuts) which had been lodged there for a very long time," and the bowels were up to 12 inches in diameter. Dr. Jensen concluded that the average patient does not know whether or not he is constipated.

Dr. John Harvey Kellogg, who lived to 91, said that we should completely eliminate the residue of each meal 15 to 18 hours after eating it. He said 90 percent of modern diseases are due to colon problems. And what is the way to eliminate your risk of colon diseases? A high-fiber, GreenSmoothieGirl diet rich in the natural anti-cancer compounds found in raw plant foods, of course. No chemotherapy, surgery, or even vitamin pill will ever be able to do what live compounds in real food, and a clean, pink, peristaltic colon, can.

Final comments on cleansing

Some people won't be ready for some of what Dr. Richard Anderson (see book reviews on GreenSmoothieGirl.com) and others who have experienced deep cleansing have to say. Some, for instance, believe that negative thoughts, emotions, and experiences are trapped in our proteins, and as mucoid plaque builds up throughout our vast lengths of intestines and colon, we retain those negatives in rather physical ways. It's theory and I find nothing that "proves" it. I rolled my eyes a bit when I first read it. But, only someone who has released all that stuff can speak to the very real spiritual and psychological power (joy, even) of letting go of decades' worth of negatives—harbored resentments and toxic anger. My first cleanse was honestly one of the singular experiences of my life: powerful, unforgettable, and wholly positive in ways that transcend the physical.

Many ancient texts speak of body cleansing, the need to fast now and then, for both physical and spiritual purification. You don't have to be a yogi to give your organs of elimination a chance to rest and repair. Over time, if you eat a 60–80 percent raw diet that includes a quart of green smoothie daily, and if you virtually eliminate processed foods and meat/dairy, you may experience slower but equally excellent results.

This is not a recommendation of any specific cleansing plan for *you*, but rather a general opinion that having a clean colon leads to improved health. Consult your health care professional about any cleanse you may be considering.

14

Making the Smoothies

Many people like to follow very specific instructions. For this purpose, I have developed the recipes in this book, all of them tested in my kitchen. However, part of the beauty of green smoothies is their free-form, creative, anything-goes nature. So, if you're already comfortable in the kitchen and a creative soul, just use the "template recipe" given here first. To be honest, it's all I ever really use. That way, I can use whatever I have on hand.

The beauty of my template recipe is it maximizes greens and minimizes fruit for the average palate. As you get off processed sugar, you may find you can tolerate and even enjoy higher proportions of greens, but most people who are open-minded about food like smoothies made with the proportions in the template recipe. For children previously raised on a processed-food diet, or for "picky eaters," you may want to start with more fruit and/or sweetener and fewer greens, and work your way to a better ratio.

Remember that the major point of the green smoothie, of course, is the greens. Putting a pinch of spinach into a fruit smoothie is better than nothing, but challenge yourself to get several servings of raw greens out of your blender adventures. If you're easily bored and don't want a similar taste every day, then use the recipes.

I like to blend the water and greens first. I do this to ensure that the greens are completely puréed, as no one appreciates a chunk of greens in what is, by definition, supposed to be smooth. (We're less likely to be offended by a chunk of banana or strawberry!) The unfrozen fruits tend to be softer, so I add them after the green purée is done. They need less blending and I don't want to oxidize them more than is necessary. I also like maximum liquid in my Total Blender to make the blending easier before adding frozen items like chunks of bananas or strawberries. Other people like to make their smoothies differently, and some blend fruit and water, and then greens. There's no "wrong" way to do it!

Remember that variety is not only the "spice of life" that makes eating fun, but it also provides a wide spectrum of nutrients. The more variety in greens and fruit (and other high-nutrition additions to your smoothies), the better! But I'm often asked something like this: "I don't like most greens, so is it okay if I just use spinach and my favorite fruits?"

The answer to that is yes, that's certainly better than nothing. However, I want to challenge you to try new things. You have available to you a huge variety of greens out there, many of which you may not be considering. You can find new ones you haven't tried before in Asian, Latin, or health food stores. We cover the nutritional properties of various greens in this book in detail but, just for review, don't forget to try more of these:

Traditional Greens/Lettuces:
- Kale
- Red chard
- Butter lettuce
- Miner's lettuce
- Arugula
- Spinach
- Napa cabbage
- Tatsoi
- Parsley
- Rainbow Swiss chard
- Endive
- Romaine
- Mache
- Vegetable amaranth
- Red cabbage
- Bok choy
- Pac choi
- Radicchio
- Swiss chard
- Escarole
- Mixed greens (mesclun)
- Celery
- Collard greens
- Green cabbage
- Yu choy
- Mizuna

Tops of root vegetables, etc.:
- Beet greens
- Turnip greens
- Grape leaves
- Kohlrabi tops
- Carrot tops
- Dandelion greens
- Mustard greens
- Jerusalem artichoke tops
- Strawberry tops (organic)
- Radish greens
- Anise/Fennel greens

Sea Vegetables:
- Arame
- Nori
- Kelp
- Kombu
- Hijiki
- Wakame
- Dulse

Weeds (Google for photos):
- Purslane
- Lambsquarter
- Morning glory
- Japanese knotweed
- Creeping Charlie

Sprouts:
- Broccoli sprouts
- Fenugreek
- Quinoa
- Bean sprouts
- Radish
- Pea greens
- Alfalfa
- Clover

Herbs:
- Mint leaves
- Lemon grass
- Bay leaves
- Tarragon leaves
- Marjoram
- Cilantro (coriander)
- Basil leaves
- Horseradish root
- Chives
- Oregano leaves

Fruits for Green Smoothies

I've never met a fruit yet that isn't great in smoothies! Use whatever is in season to save money. But my staples are bana -

nas and frozen mixed berries (both are least expensive at Costco). Bananas add a creamy texture. Frozen mixed berries make smoothies a darker color for people who revolt at the big green glass, as well as bring the sugar level down a bit and add lots of fiber. Pears are my third-favorite fruit ingredient because they're sweet and balance greens so perfectly. But you have many other options, all of which I use when those fruits are affordable and available. These are ingredients you might consider, and this list is by no means comprehensive.

Apricots	Guanabana	Pears
Apples	Grapefruit	Peaches
Bananas	Honeydew melon	Persimmons
Blackberries	Kiwi	Pineapple
Blueberries	Kumquats	Plums
Boysenberries	Lemons	Prunes
Cherries, Bing	Limes	Raspberries
Cantaloupe	Marionberries	Star fruit
Cherries, pie	Mango	Strawberries
Cranberries	Nectarines	Tangerines
Crenshaw melon	Oranges	Tangelos
Grapes	Papaya	Watermelon

Superfood Additions for Smoothies

Many health food nuts like me have a mental list of ingredients they know are nutritional powerhouses. We want to get them in our diet but often fail to do so because we don't know how or simply don't fit them into the day's menu. Green smoothies are the perfect way to do that—just toss some stuff in! Be adventurous. Use those exotic, high-impact nutrition items if you can afford them. If not, please don't worry about it—you're getting tons of fiber, vitamins, minerals, and enzymes from the simple greens and fruit combinations.

Smoothies don't have to contain expensive, exotic ingredients. But not all of the "other ingredients" discussed in this section are expensive.

See part 1 and 2 videos called "Green Smoothie 2.0" on GreenSmoothieGirl.com where I show the use of many of these superfoods in my blender.

Acai berries (pronounced "ah-sah-ee")

Acai is a very trendy health product showing up mostly in overpriced pasteurized juices sold through network marketing channels. It's native to the Amazon rainforest and, like gojis, it's off the chart in antioxidants and anthocyanins (also present in red wine), which have been studied for their heart-protecting benefits (but without the attendant health problems caused by alcohol). Like gojis, acai berries are also high in the essential fatty acids omega-6 and omega-9, and are very expensive.

If you want to spend the money, I would recommend buying the whole berries rather than concentrated juices. The juices are artificially high in sugars, even if they are natural sugars, and highly acidic as well. The nutrients may be concentrated, but pasteurized juices have no enzymes and, therefore, draw on the body's ability to manufacture them, and sugars are concentrated as well. Wherever possible, use the whole food rather than a processed version of them.

Aloe vera

Aloe vera is an inexpensive extra ingredient and something I would encourage everyone (except pregnant women, until further testing is done for that population) to use in green smoothies. I keep an aloe vera plant in my windowsill for quick and effective treatment of burns or scrapes. (You simply cut a spear from the plant, slice it in half, and rub the inner pulp on the sunburn or stovetop/curling iron burn for dramatic healing.) You can buy these plants in nurseries, and they grow wild in some very warm climates, such as in Arizona.

Aloe vera has been extensively studied for its immune-stimulating effects, and hundreds of research papers have been published documenting some very interesting benefits. One I find most interesting is the fact that it contains vitamin B12, one of the only plant-based sources of this nutrient, so adding this ingredient to smoothies can help vegans and vegetarians achieve complete nutrition. Additionally, the plant has anti-inflammatory, antibacterial, and antifungal properties. It heals ulcers and reduces asthma symptoms.

I often cut a large spear, wash it, and throw it in my green smoothie as well. Having your own plant is inexpensive, compared to the slightly processed and nutritionally inferior product you can buy in health food stores. (The juice in the jug from the health food store is still excellent nutrition—just not as powerful as a spear from the raw plant.) A small amount is best, as you can overdo this ingredient and cause too much bowel stimulation, especially if you're new to green smoothies and transitioning from a fairly typical American diet.

Avocado

Avocado adds extremely nutritious fats to your smoothie; a small amount of fat aids the body in utilizing the minerals in greens. I highly recommend adding it to smoothies for babies and children, too, or anyone who might need to gain weight. (It's not a food that will promote weight gain, but because of its high monounsaturated fat content, it's higher in calories than most green smoothie ingredients.) Avocado is one of the most perfect first foods for a baby. It's extraordinarily high in lutein, a phytonutrient that promotes strong eyesight and retards degenerative conditions of the eye. Other research shows that even short-term avocado consumption decreases total and LDL cholesterol.

Bee pollen

Bee pollen has been a fascination of European researchers for a long time. The dust from the stamen of blossoming plants collected from bees is fairly well documented to improve a lot of things most of us care about. First of all, it increases your energy throughout the day and stamina for physical activity—it's a powerhouse nutritionally, with 35 percent protein.

Studies suggest it has natural weight-loss properties that have been mimicked chemically in various weight-loss drug remedies. Bee pollen not only stimulates metabolism, but also suppresses appetite naturally. It slows aging and prevents cancerous tumors from developing.

It also contains a gonadotropic sex hormone and contributes to improved sexual performance and reduction of PMS symptoms. Perhaps, most interestingly, it may prevent seasonal allergies, like eating raw honey allegedly does, but in a more direct way and without the blood sugar impact.

If you can, buy it collected from multiple sources instead of one source; this makes a better product. Bee pollen is a fantastic ingredient to add to a green smoothie. At the time of this writing, I like to get it from All Star Health on Amazon because (a) the price is good, (b) it's very fresh and not dry like other sources, and (c) they collect it from around the U.S. so it's not just one geographic area's bees, which I feel is best for allergy prevention.

The occasional person will have an allergic reaction to bee pollen, so try just a few granules your first day, and increase a little bit daily for a few days until you're sure you're not reacting to it. A good amount to get daily is one teaspoon, either plain or in your smoothie.

I feel more comfortable recommending bee pollen to you than other products commonly marketed, such as royal bee jelly (which is fed to the queen bee to make her large and fertile) or bee propolis (the resin from tree buds that bees collect). More data has been collected on the benefits of the pollen.

Brewer's (nutritional) yeast

Brewer's or "nutritional" yeast is grown on barley, and it's often used as a supplement, especially by nursing mothers to increase milk supply. It's high in protein and is also extremely rich in B vitamins. It has been linked to the reduction of symptoms of diabetes, eczema, constipation, and hypoglycemia.

It's also one of very few plant sources of B12. Vegetarian lifestyles are often criticized for their low intake of vitamin B12, and while vegetarians may not actually be suffering from low B12 (depending on which study you look at), using aloe vera and nutritional yeast are good ways to address that if you're avoiding all red meat.

Cayenne pepper

Cayenne pepper has long been used not only for a "heat" spice, but also for the medicinal purpose of opening the arteries and preventing cardiac events. Dr. Christopher famously gave people a cup of "cayenne tea" (one teaspoon in hot water) after cardiac events and said they would always be up and around immediately because it works faster than any pill. Cayenne is well known to herbalists for its ability to accelerate and intensify the effects of other herbs. It'll add heat and interesting flavor to your smoothies, and also open your blood vessels, improving circulation; in addition, it's anti-nausea, antiallergy, and anti-constipation. Research has shown that cayenne also has the ability to kill cancer cells on contact.

Chia seed

With so much focus on essential fatty acids (EFAs) and omega fats, the chia seed is a standout because it's 40 percent omega-6 oil. So many people are taking EFA supplements that this whole food, with its high omega 6:3 ratio, is very attractive.

Chia seeds absorb ten times their weight in water, so they're good thickeners when soaked. They also give you a sense of fullness, a great aid in weight loss. Some think they absorb some food calories as well, making them a diet helper in more ways than one. They slow the conversion of carbohydrates into sugars and, therefore, help maintain stable blood sugar levels, great for everyone, especially diabetics.

You can sprinkle chia seeds on anything as they have a neutral flavor, and unlike flaxseed, they're digestible without needing to be ground. But, unlike flax, they're quite expensive.

Chocolate, raw

Organic chocolate bars and acai berries are often marketed together. (And no wonder—it's a delicious, if expensive, combination.)

Dark chocolate has been touted in recent years for its very high Oxygen Radical Absorbance Capacity (ORAC) score, which means high antioxidants and consequent ability to protect against free radicals that age us and cause disease. Some people are confused by this and think that chocolate products found in health food stores are, then, high-nutrition items. Most products, even those marketed to health nuts like you and me, have sweeteners added (sometimes even processed sweeteners) and are cooked to eliminate the benefits of

enzymes. They also have additives like alkali that are not beneficial and can even be destructive. One network-marketed
candy claims to be a health food, costs $60 per pound, is arti-
ficially sweetened, and isn't even organic. You can spend $10 a
pound for raw dark chocolate bars in the health food stores,
and that's still a pricey treat.

The one type of chocolate I'd advocate you adding to your
green smoothies is raw, organic cacao nibs or powdered cacao.
You can find these products online (Amazon is probably the
cheapest) or in a health food store. They make lovely treats
and smoothies when you add agave and blend them with
frozen berries in a smoothie (coconut milk or coconut meat or
almond milk are also good additions, making fantastic dessert-
like concoctions in your Total Blender). But raw chocolate
products are extremely expensive.

Coconut oil, liquid, or meat

Raw coconut is prized for its antibacterial, antimicrobial,
antifungal, and antiviral properties. Dr. Bruce Fife's *The Coconut Oil Miracle* effectively covers the research on this rather
miraculous food, showing how a fat is not always a fat. Non-
Westernized Pacific Islanders have ideal height-weight ratios
and virtually no heart disease; they're some of the most beautiful people on the planet. Their diet relies so heavily on
coconut that, despite it being a "saturated" fat, the Pacific-
Islander indigenous diet is sometimes as high as 60 percent
calories from fat, with extremely low rates of overweight people. They don't suffer from anxiety and depression, and they
don't get cancer.

Coconut meat is a great raw dessert recipe ingredient that
I use a lot in *12 Steps to Whole Foods* (on GreenSmoothieGirl.

com). If you buy the young Thai coconuts, found most inexpensively in Asian markets, you can drain the liquid and scrape the meat out—I have a YouTube video showing how to do this most easily. You can certainly add coconut meat to your green smoothies, but since the meat will thicken the smoothie considerably, add extra water (or coconut liquid).

Coconut liquid is low in fat, tastes delicious, and is so electrolyte-rich that it's now sold in boxes with straws, in the refrigerated section in health food stores with the sports drinks. It's a perfect drink for an athlete to balance electrolytes, so much better than commercial sports drinks that contain lots of chemicals plus artificial sweeteners and colors. It's also high in minerals, and preeminent raw foodist David Wolfe calls it a "blood transfusion" because of the way it closely parallels human blood chemistry and nourishes us so exactly.

Coconut oil is a power food as well, harnessing the antiviral and antibacterial properties and fat-burning power of the coconut. If you add coconut oil to your green smoothies, blend it in well with the non-refrigerated and non-frozen items first. It becomes solid at 76 degrees, so you may have tiny solid particles of the oil in your smoothie if you don't incorporate it well. Dr. Fife recommends a couple of tablespoons daily in the diet for the average adult, and/or absorbed into the bloodstream by using it on the skin and lips as a moisturizer.

Flax oil

If you don't know how to get flax oil in your diet, adding a few tablespoons to a blender container full of smoothie is easy. Minerals from greens are absorbed better when eaten with some fats, so putting flax oil in your green smoothie is a great idea. You'll never even notice it. A tablespoon daily is a good dosage for an adult to avoid inflammatory ailments; it also protects healthy cell membranes needed to keep toxic elements out but allow nutrients in. Flax oil has wide-ranging benefits uncovered in research in the past decade, involving the immune, circulatory, reproductive, cardiovascular, and nervous systems. It's rich in essential fatty acids, including the rare omega-6 and omega-9 nutrients that your body cannot manufacture itself and must receive from outside sources.

Using flax oil, you can avoid taking fish oil with all its attendant risks (fish being tainted with mercury and other pollutants). Flax has 80 times more lignans than the next-highest food. These compounds which cut your risk of breast and colon cancers dramatically. Research connects flax to reduction of PMS symptoms, improvement in multiple sclerosis treatment, and reduction in allergies, arthritis, and diabetes, as well as eczema, asthma, and loss of eyesight. It increases fat burning and allows you to recover from sprains and muscle fatigue more quickly.

You should never heat flax oil, which damages its nutritional properties, and you must purchase it refrigerated and use it very fresh, as it becomes rancid in only a month or two. This is one of the more expensive ingredients you can add to smoothies. If you prefer, you can grind a small amount of flaxseed instead. This is inexpensive, but the whole seed is mucilaginous, thereby making your smoothie thicker and bulkier, so if you add ground flaxseed instead of oil, you may want to add more water to compensate. Use freshly ground flaxseed, as it oxidizes and becomes rancid quickly once ground. You can use your high-power blender, or a small ten-dollar electric coffee grinder from any store such as Target or Walmart.

Ginger

Ginger is an ingredient I add to my smoothies almost daily. The most inexpensive place I find to buy it is Asian stores, and I always pick some up when I stop by for my cases of young Thai coconuts. The unpeeled ginger "roots" last a few weeks in the fridge. (At the Asian market, I also look through their interesting greens selection and take home some cabbages for variety in green smoothies.)

Fresh ginger is not actually a root, but rather an underground stem. You peel the brown outer layer off and add an inch or two, or more, to any smoothie. It adds a lovely flavor, but it also has powerful anti-inflammatory, digestive-function strengthening, and anti-nausea properties. It's a great natural remedy for motion sickness, morning sickness, and intestinal gas. If someone struggles with feeling nauseous while starting a green-smoothie habit, I recommend adding as much ginger as you can. It's a warming herb that helps stimulate blood circulation and promotes decongestion, and it can help knock down a fever.

Goji berries

Goji berries are an interesting food because they've been consumed regularly by the Earth's longest-living people for at least the past 1,700 years, as well as used medicinally. The berries are 13 percent protein, unheard of for a fruit, and they will increase the protein ratio of almost any green smoothie.

They also have several B vitamins and vitamin E, also rare in fruits, 18 amino acids, and possibly more antioxidants than any other food ever studied (though dark chocolate is a competitor). Remember that antioxidants scavenge free radicals, literally mopping up those little cancer-causing destroyers in the body. Many of the compounds found in abundance in the goji berry are so newly researched that we're only just beginning to understand how these nutrients cause increased disease resistance.

Goji berries are very expensive, up to $20 per pound. Some of my local readers and I have planted goji plants, which do well in cold winter climates, since the indigenous climates it originates in (such as Tibet) are cold and mountainous as well. The bushes become fairly large and grow quickly.

Lemon peel

Lemon peel is another ingredient I add almost daily. I often buy a large bag of lemons at Costco, or I bring them home from California or Arizona when I visit. I freeze the lemon juice in ice cube trays for use in guacamole, raw desserts, and homemade salad dressings. (Many recipes are found in *12 Steps to Whole Foods* on GreenSmoothieGirl.com.) But I don't throw the lemon peels away! I cut them in eighths (having washed the lemons well first) and freeze them. Every day I get a piece of lemon peel out of the freezer and toss it in my smoothie. It's a bit bitter, so it's best when stevia or agave is added to the mix to offset the bitterness.

With its potent flavonoids, lemon peel has been linked by research to preventing and killing skin cancers. As a teenager and young adult, I laid out in the sun for hours, nearly daily, from April to October. I was always brown, but only after burning many times. I'm more careful now, but still love the sun and never use sunscreen. The only reason I can explain why I look younger than I am and have no skin cancer, despite being a fair-skinned redhead, is my excellent nutrition and near-daily use of lemon peel!

Kelp and dulse

If you don't mind the seaweedy taste of sea vegetables like kelp and dulse, use these high-impact foods in your blender. Just a little bit is enough, and they're more thyroid nourishing than any other food. So if you're hypothyroid (as about 25 percent of women are in America, many of them undiagnosed), consider getting one or both of these foods in your daily diet. Green smoothies are an easy way to do that. Those who suffer with low energy and slow metabolism often have low thyroid problems. (And diagnosing it can be difficult, involving full-panel blood testing done by a hormone clinic, examining the interplay of several different variables.) Taking a thyroid hormone, especially synthetic drugs such as Synthroid and Cytomel, causes disease risk and can burn out the thyroid even more over time. Sea vegetables nourish and support the thyroid rather than jab and poke it (and thus wearing it out over time), like drugs do, to make it perform.

Maca root

Maca is a very trendy product from an ancient Peruvian food. It's a root related to turnips and radishes because it's been linked by research to endocrine health and a healthy libido. It's also said to improve energy levels throughout the day. So the aphrodisiac is used in South America to boost performance in a variety of areas. In powdered form, it's an easy addition to green smoothies.

Pomegranate juice

Pomegranate juice is another very hot product because of a few studies linking it to slowing growth of prostate cancer and arthritis, and reduction of breast and skin cancer. It's been linked to improvement of several cardiovascular measurements, including thinning the blood and improving blood flow, lowering LDS cholesterol, and increasing HDL ("good") cholesterol.

I'd prefer to see people use the whole fruit, which is available in the winter. You peel away the red outer peel and the inner white membranes to harvest the seeds, which look exactly like rubies. It's a little more labor intensive to take apart a pomegranate than to prepare other fruit. However, it's fun for children because the fruit is so beautiful and a bit of a treasure hunt.

All juices are concentrated, with high natural sugar content, and also quite acidic. The whole fruit (while lower in vitamin and mineral concentrations) achieves the same benefit of pomegranate juice without the downside of a product that lacks live enzymes and is high in sugar.

Sprouts

Sprouts are so easy to grow, yet most people don't eat them at all. They're living things, and they're little enzyme-packed powerhouses. When the seed, nut, or legume sprouts, all the enzyme potential is unlocked to go into that burst of energy that becomes a plant. You have the opportunity, at that unparalleled nutritional level, to steal that nutrition for yourself. Sprouts have the capacity to dramatically reduce your reliance on the body's need to manufacture enzymes and, consequently, steal from metabolic processes. When you eat them, you're oxygenating your body and starving cancer cells— think of eating sprouts as the very opposite of eating sugar and other toxic foods that nourish cancer and make your body a host for all kinds of immediate and future problems.

They're great on sandwiches, and I add them to granola I serve my children every morning. But many people have a hard time finding ways to sneak them into their diet, and blending them into a smoothie is easy and painless. Just add them as part of the greens portion of the recipe.

I would not use sprouted nuts or large seeds like pumpkin and sunflower in green smoothies (unless you're using "greened" sunflower sprouts—when the seed is grown into greens). Those large nut and seed sprouts will make a smoothie heavy and thick. I'd stick to the smaller seeds like clover, alfalfa, and fenugreek for green smoothie ingredients.

Wheat germ, raw

Raw wheat germ is extremely high in vitamin E and the B vitamins, so this is a great ingredient for women with PMS or menopausal symptoms. In addition, eating it prevents some birth defects, according to research. It'll help you achieve glossy hair, pretty skin, and strong nails. It adds a nutty flavor and thickness to the smoothie, so you'll want to add extra water when using this ingredient. It's a great way to add fiber to your diet, promoting colonic peristalsis and avoiding constipation and diseases such as colon cancer.

However, raw wheat germ goes rancid very quickly. Buy it in bulk at your health food store if you trust that the store has good product turnover and buys fresh product often. Taste it before using, and if it has an even slightly rancid taste, don't use it. Store it in the fridge for no more than a couple of months, preferably in an airtight container to slow oxidation.

Wheatgrass juice (fresh or powdered)

Wheatgrass was first famously studied and used extensively by Ann Wigmore, founder of Optimum Health Institute and a pioneer of many therapies still used now, 50 years later, in natural healing. She wrote *The Wheatgrass Book*, documenting its megapowerful healing properties.

If I had cancer, the first thing I'd do is begin growing, juicing, and drinking wheatgrass daily. Nothing compares to it nutritionally for oxygenating and healing. I have juiced wheatgrass in a few periods of my life (including an early pregnancy, which may have been part of my current problem with it), and I'd continue the habit if it weren't simply the most awful-tasting thing on this planet. Not everyone agrees with my assessment, fortunately, so give it a try.

In the event you can't stomach the fresh juice, more and more companies are dehydrating the juice under 118 degrees and selling it as a powder. While I find this to be too much in a green smoothie, some people like it. I prefer to see people add this ingredient to water to alkalize their cells and energize them throughout the day, since your green smoothie already provides many of the ingredients concentrated in wheatgrass.

Generally speaking, wheatgrass is juiced and the remaining grass discarded because its fiber is not digestible by the human stomach. The juicers we used ten years ago were not efficient at getting the juice from the grass, which is digestible only by a four-chambered stomach such as that found in a cow. However, completely liquefied wheatgrass, such as that which occurs in a high-power blender, may render unnecessary the expensive, labor-intensive, and messy process we used to go through with specialized wheatgrass juicers.

Yogurt or kefir

Yogurt or kefir, particularly homemade, adds a creamy, smooth texture to smoothies. You can learn more about this topic in *12 Steps to Whole Foods,* including how to make them at home inexpensively and easily. Kefir and yogurt are the only animal products I actively promote, as their proteins are predigested and broken down for easy utilization by the body, unlike other animal proteins.

Even more importantly, they contribute to a healthy gastrointestinal tract by populating it with good micro-organisms that are your main defense against bacterial infections and other harmful micro-organisms. Most people have 10:1 bad microorganisms to good, and the ratio should be reversed for a healthy colon. The best way to address this is to eat yogurt or kefir daily and avoid foods (like dairy, meat, and processed foods) that feed the bad bacteria.

If you're going to purchase commercial yogurt or kefir, organic is better, and buy plain flavor rather than the excessively sugar-sweetened vanilla and other flavors. Goat yogurt is nutritionally superior to dairy (cow's milk) products. It's not mucus forming and is easier to digest, due to a smaller fat molecule that permeates semi-permeable human membranes without triggering the body's defense mechanism to flush out with mucus. People do not experience "lactose intolerance" with goat's milk products, and many who are lactose intolerant with regular milk do not experience those symptoms with dairy yogurt.

List of Superfood Additions

Regardless of the recipe you use for your smoothies, you may wish to keep the following list on your fridge or inside a cabinet to remind yourself to put in your daily smoothie a few ingredients with properties you're interested in. That way, you remember to use these specialty ingredients you've purchased before they expire.

- Acai berries
- Aloe vera (bottled or fresh)
- Avocado

- Bee pollen
- Brewer's (nutritional) yeast
- Cayenne pepper (ground)
- Chia seed
- Chocolate, raw (powder or nibs)

- Coconut liquid or meat
- Coconut oil (virgin, organic)
- Flax oil (refrigerated, fresh)
- Flaxseed

- Ginger (fresh, peeled)
- Goji berries
- Herbs, fresh (dill, mint, etc.)
- Lemon peel
- Lime peel
- Maca
- Pomegranate juice
- Royal bee jelly or propolis
- Sprouts of any seed
- Wheat germ, raw
- Wheatgrass juice
- Yogurt or kefir

Sweeteners for Smoothies, and Sugar Restrictions

I have two favorite sweeteners for green smoothies, stevia and agave, plus a few others I use occasionally.

Stevia

If you're diabetic, hypoglycemic, or trying to cut down on sugar, using stevia as your smoothie sweetener (or use no sweetener at all) is wise. Stevia is 100 times sweeter than sugar, but it's derived from an herb and is natural (though processors do add fillers to the powdered versions and a base to the liquid versions), so you can use ¼ to ½ tsp. to sweeten a full blender of smoothie. You can purchase stevia either powdered or in liquid drops at any health food store.

In Asia, stevia has been widely used and well known for decades, although it has not been studied in clinical trials.

Many forces, including governmental ones, conspired to keep stevia out of the hands of American consumers for many years, even banning it from the shelves of stores selling food. This was not because of any consumer complaints about side effects (no side effects of stevia have been documented as of this writing), but because of the monopolistic chokehold that the manufacturers of the artificial sweetener aspartame (Nutra-Sweet) had on the American food industry.

I believe the erosion of aspartame's power, as it has begun to give way to Splenda (much like saccharin gave way to aspartame many years ago), created the opportunity for stevia to become accepted in the Western hemisphere. Aspartame's current decline can be directly attributed to the fact that, of over 4,000 food additives approved by the FDA, aspartame has more health-related complaints than all the other food additives put together! Aspartame is a deadly excitotoxin linked to neurological problems, including seizures, cancer, and many other problems.

If you don't like the taste of stevia in the form you purchase it, you may wish to try another kind (powdered, liquid drops, flavored drops, etc.) or brand. I don't notice an aftertaste, but some who use stevia say they do.

Agave Nectar

My second-favorite smoothie-sweetening option nutritionally (and my favorite option taste-wise) is to use raw, organic agave nectar, derived from cactus plants. I've compared properties of light and dark varieties and don't see a big advantage to either one nutritionally, nor do I notice a significant taste difference. The big advantage of using agave rather than other sweeteners is that it has one-third the glycemic index of sugar and honey. It's a light syrup with a pleasant, neutral flavor that you won't notice, and it's sweeter than sugar. You can purchase it online or in health food stores, or inexpensively by the gallon or case.

Agave has gotten a bad rap lately, as allegations have been made that Mexican companies sometimes cut high-fructose corn syrup into agave. Madhava is a good brand, and they process their "raw" agave under 118 degrees. Some brands that advertise to be raw probably are not. So, if you can, use a brand that clearly states its commitment to cold processing, since that's how enzymes are preserved.

Dates

Dates are an ancient food very high in magnesium and calcium. As a whole, raw food, they're an excellent sweetener and will have less impact on blood sugar. I buy them chopped and rolled in oat flour only because they cost about half as much that way (you can rinse the oat flour off if you want). Use an equivalent amount of dates to whatever is called for in the recipe for agave (a 1:1 ratio).

Honey

Honey is very concentrated and sweetens a green smoothie very well. The upside to this sweetener is, if used raw, it may have the ability to decrease or eliminate your seasonal allergies. Regarding raw honey, some theorize that the cross-pollination done by local bees provides a type of homeopathic remedy. I tried this myself when I first read about it and did not have seasonal allergies ever again after using small amounts of local, raw product. The product is not technically considered vegan since "animals" (bees) can be harmed in the production.

The downside to honey is that it's very high on the glycemic index, which means it provides a jolt to your blood sugar comparable to sugar and corn syrup. Honey is much higher in nutrients, of course, but for those with blood sugar issues, it's best avoided. When you use it, do so in small amounts.

Maple Syrup

Maple syrup is never technically raw, but its nutrient content is certainly much higher than sugar or corn syrup, and because of the pleasant flavor, many raw foodists favor it as a sweetener. It's also expensive. Grade B is more unprocessed and, therefore, better than Grade A. Use maple syrup in a pinch, but keep in mind that it's a concentrated sweetener that has a relatively high impact on your blood sugar, so agave and stevia are your best options.

15

Recipes

If you're new to green smoothies or are feeling a little wary of what your concoctions might taste like, start with my Template Recipe below. If you're feeling adventurous, know that I've tried to experiment with almost every kind of green edible in these recipes. If you have an unusual "leafy green" in your possession and don't know what to do with it, go to the index of this book and look it up. Chances are it's an ingredient in one of the following recipes!

Robyn's Green Smoothie Template Recipe

Makes 8 cups of 100 percent raw smoothie.

Tips: For beginners and those trying to convert children, consider using *less* greens and *more* fruit (especially berries and bananas) in the beginning, gradually working up to a 50/50 ratio as described here. In this transition phase, use just the mild flavors like spinach, kale, collards, and chard. With kids, consider using only spinach the first few days, then sneak in chard, collards, and kale gradually. Add other savory or bitter greens only when your family is "expert" in green smoothies! Add a bit more water if you feel the smoothie is too thick.

Put 2½ cups filtered water in a high-power blender.

Optionally, add:

> ½ tsp. stevia (herbal sweetener) or ¼ cup raw, organic agave nectar (low glycemic index)
>
> ¼ whole lemon, including peel (anti-skin cancer, high in flavonoids)
>
> 2–3 Tbsp. fresh, refrigerated flax oil (omega-3 rich oil)

Gradually add until, briefly puréed, the mixture comes up to the 5-cup line (or less if you're "converting"):

> ¾ to 1 lb. raw, washed greens, added up to 5½ cup line:
>
> spinach, chard, kale, collards are your mainstays
>
> turnip, mustard, dandelion greens, arugula—use more sparingly, as they're spicy or bitter
>
> lettuces and beet greens are also good—use freely
>
> try avocado or cabbage or 1–2 stalks celery

Purée the greens mixture for 90 seconds, until very smooth.

Gradually add fruit until the container is very full (8 cups or more), blend 90 seconds or until smooth:

> 1–2 bananas to add a creamy texture and sweetness
>
> 1–2 cups frozen mixed berries (tastes wonderful and makes the smoothie purple rather than green)
>
> any other fruit to taste: our favorites are pears and peaches, but also apples, oranges, apricots, cantaloupes (with seeds—very high in antioxidants!), mangoes, pineapples, anything!

The more frozen fruit you add, the tastier your smoothie will be, and a high-power blender can handle it! You can save your smoothie in the fridge for up to two days—just shake well before drinking.

Laura's Little-or-No-Fruit Green Smoothie

Some of you want to skip the fruit in your smoothie altogether. Maybe you're trying to cut out sugars (even unrefined fruit sugar), or you're on the candida diet, or you're diabetic or highly hypoglycemic. If so, try this all-green smoothie that is both highly edible as well as nutrition-packed and low in sugar. It also has some necessary and nutritious fat in the form of avocado.

My former university student Laura spent seven years of her adolescence and young adult life in bed with serious health issues. She doesn't do well with sugar of any kind and devised this green smoothie that's highly alkaline and low in sugar. This recipe is for die-hards only—the type who'll drink anything for health, regardless of taste. That said, it tastes better than you'd think!

    1 avocado
    1 large cucumber
    2 cups spinach
    2 large leaves collard greens
    2 leaves black kale
    2–3 lemons, juice only (to taste)
    1 ½ cups water
    optional: a few slices of Gala apples
    Purée well and enjoy.

Important Notes before You Use the Following Recipes

The remaining recipes in this book have a yield of 6 pints, and are most easily made in a large (96-ounce) container. (The template recipe above will fit in a Vita-Mix or the smaller 64-ounce container that comes with your Blendtec.) If you have the smaller, 64-ounce container that comes with your machine, you can still use these large-batch recipes (see Note 2 about why you may want to consider doing so), but you'll fill up your container before adding all the fruit. Just blend as much of the ingredient list that fits in the container until smooth, and pour half of the mixture out into your glass jars. Then add the rest of the fruit, blend again, and pour the remainder into the jars. Put a lid on the jars and shake well.

If you prefer smaller batches, just cut the recipes in half for a yield of approximately three pints. I developed these large-batch, three-quart recipes for a family's needs, or for one person doing the three-day detox plan. At my house, I use this batch for a quart daily for me, and a pint daily for each of my four children. I maximize how much I can get out of the blender and fill the container very full.

Keep in mind that if three quarts are too much for you, you can save green smoothies for the next day. (That's as long as they'll last, though. By the third day, they'll have lost a lot of nutrition and will taste funky, too.)

I highly recommend owning the largest container (96-ounce) for the Blendtec and making these large batches, even for a single person. A single person can drink a quart that day, save a quart for the next day, and freeze a quart for a third day. This way, you're cutting your time and effort by two-thirds for the same benefit. It'll make a big difference in your ability to get excellent nutrition within your busy schedule. Instead of spending ten minutes in the kitchen daily, a single person can spend ten minutes every *third* day. Just remember to get the frozen smoothie out several hours before you want to use it, and shake it well before drinking.

I use spinach in most of these recipes. One reason is that it's not only high in protein, but also outstanding in virtually all nutritional measures. A more practical reason, though, is that it's easy to have spinach on hand. Costco sells huge, 2.5-

pound bags of spinach at the time of this writing for $3.95, as well as more expensive tubs of organic baby spinach. Using lots of spinach helps keep smoothie costs low. (Use other greens for taste as well as that all-important vitamin and mineral variety.) So, considering simplicity for my readers, I include spinach as the last green you add to a recipe to achieve the maximum greens-to-fruit ratio.

Aloe and Apple

2¾ cups water/ice

2 large spears of fresh aloe vera, cut from the plant (or ¼ cup bottled)

4 large collard leaves

Spinach, added until mixture reaches 6-cup line

1–2 inches fresh ginger, peeled

2 large Granny Smith apples

2 bananas, frozen in chunks

3 cups frozen blueberries

½ tsp. stevia

Blend first 4 ingredients until smooth. Add fruit and stevia and blend until smooth. Serve immediately for best results, or refrigerate up to 24 hours in glass jars and shake well before serving.

Arugula Arame Attack

3 cups water/ice

2 large handfuls arugula

¼ cup arame or wakame, or 1 raw nori sheet (Asian sea vegetable)

Spinach, added until mixture reaches 6-cup line

2 cups pineapple, preferably frozen in chunks

2 bananas, frozen in chunks

2 cups frozen blueberries, blackberries, or mixed berries

1 apple or pear

½ tsp. stevia

Blend first 4 ingredients until smooth. Add fruit and stevia and blend until smooth. Serve immediately for best results, or refrigerate up to 24 hours in glass jars and shake well before serving.

Asian Green Smoothie

You can experiment with a wide variety of Asian greens, sprouts, and cabbages in your smoothies by going to your local Asian market. Ingredients tend to be inexpensive in these small markets, as well.

2¼ cups water/ice

8 cups loose bok choy and yu choy (coarsely chopped)

1 cup Chinese celery

1–2 cups bean sprouts

4 tangelos

2 bananas, frozen in chunks

½ tsp. stevia

4 cups frozen mixed berries

Blend first 3 ingredients until smooth. Add remaining ingredients and purée until smooth and serve immediately (best, as sprouts oxidize and lose nutrition quickly when blended), or pour in glass jars and refrigerate for up to 24 hours.

Beet Blast

Beets are a good way to change the color of a smoothie radically for those averse to green. This recipe is a good starter for children who need a sweeter, milder smoothie to begin converting to smoothies as a way of life. This is a good winter smoothie, and I leave some beets overwintered in the garden to pull in January or February, rather than pay grocery store prices.

3¼ cups water/ice

1 medium beet, washed well and quartered

¼ of a medium green cabbage, cut in chunks

Spinach, added until mixture reaches 6-cup line

2 Tbsp. honey

2 apples (Cameo, Jonathan, Jonagold, or Gala)

2 bananas, frozen in chunks

2 cups pineapple, frozen in chunks

½ tsp. ground nutmeg

Blend first 4 ingredients for 60 seconds, then add remaining ingredients and blend until very smooth. Serve immediately, or refrigerate for up to 24 hours in glass jars and shake well before serving.

Big Black Cabbage Cocktail

3 cups water/ice

4 cups black cabbage

Spinach, added until mixture reaches 6-cup line

¼ cup raw, organic agave

2 pears

2 bananas

8 apricots, pits removed (or equivalent amount of frozen mixed fruit)

Blend first 3 ingredients until smooth. Add remaining ingredients and blend until smooth. Serve immediately, or refrigerate for up to 24 hours in glass jars and shake well before serving.

Black Kale Blackberry Brew

2¾ cups water/ice

2 stalks celery

5 large leaves black (lacinato) kale

¼ whole lemon

2 Tbsp. flax oil

2–4 Tbsp. raw, organic agave

Spinach, added until mixture reaches 6-cup line

2 cups chopped fresh pineapple (optionally frozen)

2 cups blackberries

2 bananas, frozen in chunks

Blend first 7 ingredients until smooth. Add fruit and blend until smooth. Serve immediately, or refrigerate for up to 24 hours in glass jars and shake well before serving.

Blended Salad

Many modern health complaints make eating a salad very difficult for those who suffer from them. If you like salad but can't tolerate the chewing, this recipe may be helpful for you. It makes one serving.

1 very large handful spinach

1 tomato

⅛ to ¼ red onion

½ avocado or 1 Tbsp. extra virgin olive oil

¼ zucchini or yellow squash

A few sprigs of cilantro (optional)

1 Tbsp. lemon juice

Water to achieve desired consistency

pinch of sea salt and freshly ground pepper to taste

Blend all ingredients until smooth, using minimal olive oil and water to achieve a consistency for blending. Eat with a spoon, or thin out with water to drink.

Broccoli Blitz

A good winter smoothie, and good for getting broccoli into your day, if you're like me and don't love eating it raw.

2¾ cup water/ice

¼ cup raw, organic agave

2 cups of broccoli (florets and/or stems), or broccoli rabe (found in Italian or Asian markets)

Spinach, added until mixture reaches 5-cup line

2 oranges, peeled and quartered

2 cups pineapple, chopped

2 bananas, frozen in chunks

2 cups frozen mixed berries

Blend first 4 ingredients until smooth. Add fruit and blend again until smooth. Serve immediately, or refrigerate for up to 24 hours in glass jars and shake well before serving.

Brussels Blaster

I have hated cooked Brussels sprouts since childhood. Here's a way to get their excellent, anti-cancer, cruciferous nutrition in your diet without cooking the enzymes out, and not even notice they're there.

3 cups water/ice

12 Brussels sprouts

Spinach, added until mixture reaches 6-cup line

1 yellow grapefruit, peeled

3 cups frozen mixed berries

2 bananas, frozen in chunks

1 apple

½ cup raw, organic agave

Blend first 3 ingredients until smooth. Add remaining ingredients and blend until smooth. Serve immediately, or refrigerate for up to 24 hours in glass jars and shake well before serving.

Butterhead Brew

Butterhead, Bibb, and Boston are different names for the same lettuce variety.

2¾ cups water/ice

1 head Butterhead, Bibb, or Boston lettuce, washed

½ cup clover/radish/alfalfa/fenugreek sprouts (any combination of those
   small seeds)

Spinach, added until mixture reaches 6-cup line

¼ cup raw, organic agave

2 bananas, frozen in chunks

2 oranges

2 cups frozen blueberries

2 cups frozen fruit medley or other fruit

Soak ¼ cup of seeds overnight, strain, and allow to sit another 12–24
hours, draining several times a day. Blend the first 4 ingredients well. Add agave
and fruit and blend again until smooth. Serve immediately (as sprouts oxidize
quickly).

Cabbage Cool-Aid

2¾ cups water/ice

Green cabbage, added until mixture reaches 6-cup line (yu choy or bok
   choy works, too)

4 cups frozen mixed berries

2 bananas, frozen in chunks

2 large tart apples

¼ cup raw, organic agave

Blend first 2 ingredients until smooth. Add fruit and agave and blend until
smooth. Serve immediately for best results, or refrigerate up to 24 hours in glass
jars and shake well before serving.

Carrot Top Concoction

2¾ cups water/ice

Carrot greens from 6 carrots

Spinach, added until mixture reaches 6-cup line

½ tsp. stevia

2 tart-sweet apples (Jonathan, Gala, Cameo, etc.)

2 oranges

1 banana

1–2 cups frozen berries

Blend first 3 ingredients for 1–2 minutes, then add remaining ingredients and blend until smooth. Serve immediately, or refrigerate for up to 24 hours in glass jars and shake well before serving.

Chia Choice

3¼ cups water/ice

1 Tbsp. chia seeds

Red leaf lettuce and/or chard leaves (with stems), blended into mixture to
    6-cup line

½ tsp. stevia

4 black plums, pits cut out

2 bananas, frozen in chunks

3 cups frozen berries

Optional: dash of hot sauce

Blend first 3 ingredients until smooth. Add all other ingredients and blend well. Serve immediately, or refrigerate in glass jars for up to 24 hours and shake well before serving.

Cranapple Yogurt Crave

A good winter choice, as all these ingredients are available November to March.

2½ cups water/ice

1 cup yogurt

2 leaves chard, including stems

2 leaves collards, including stems

Spinach, added until mixture reaches 6.5-cup line

⅓ cup raw, organic agave

2 cups cranberries

2 cups blueberries

1 banana, frozen in chunks

3 Cameo apples

Blend first 6 ingredients until smooth. Add remaining ingredients and blend again until smooth. Serve immediately, or refrigerate for up to 24 hours in glass jars and shake well before serving.

Dandelion Delight

4 cups dandelion greens, coarsely chopped (wild/unsprayed, or found in
    health food stores)

½ tsp. stevia

¼ cup frozen orange juice (freshly squeezed and frozen in ice cube trays—
    2 large ice cubes is ¼ cup)

Spinach, added and blended to the 6-cup line

2 oranges

2 bananas, frozen in chunks

¼ whole lemon

Frozen berries added until container is very full

Blend first 4 ingredients until smooth. Add fruit and blend until smooth.
Serve immediately, or refrigerate for up to 24 hours in glass jars and shake well before serving.

Dilly Summer Drink

2¾ cups water and ice

¹/₃ cup fresh dill weed

4 cups mesclun (mixed spring greens)

Spinach, added until mixture reaches 6-cup line

½ tsp. stevia

¹/₈ whole lemon

4 nectarines, pits removed

2 bananas

2 cups frozen mixed berries

Blend first 4 ingredients until smooth. Add remaining ingredients and blend until smooth. Serve immediately, or refrigerate for up to 24 hours and shake well before serving.

Endive Energy Express

2¾ cups water/ice

Spinach, added until mixture reaches 4-cup line

Curly endive, added and blended up to 6-cup line

¼ cup raw, organic agave

3 cups frozen mixed berries

4 clementines

2 bananas, frozen in chunks

Blend first 3 ingredients well. Add agave and fruit and blend until smooth. Serve immediately, or refrigerate for up to 24 hours in glass jars and shake well before serving.

Everything + The Kitchen Sink Garden Smoothie

2¾ cups water/ice

4 cups radish, carrot, strawberry, and/or beet tops, washed very well

1 cup weeds like purslane, dandelion, morning glory, or lambsquarter

Spinach, added until mixture reaches 6-cup line

½ tsp stevia

3 cups frozen mixed-fruit blend

2 bananas, frozen in chunks

2 cups frozen mixed berries

Blend first 4 ingredients until very smooth. Add stevia and fruit and blend until smooth. Serve immediately, or refrigerate for up to 24 hours in glass jars and shake well before serving.

Glorious Green Leaf

2¾ cups water/ice

1–2 heads green leaf lettuce (or added up to 6-cup line when blended)

1–2 inches fresh ginger, peeled

⅛ to ¼ whole lemon

¼ cup raw, organic agave

2 cups pineapple, frozen in chunks

2 oranges, peeled

2 bananas, frozen in chunks

2 cups frozen mixed berries

Blend first 3 ingredients until smooth. Add fruit and agave and blend until smooth. Serve immediately for best results, or refrigerate up to 24 hours in glass jars and shake well before serving.

Gobs of Goji

This is an easy smoothie to make in the winter because all these ingredients are available in stores, even in cold climates.

Goji berries, native to the Himalayas and Tibet, are a secret of longevity for some of the world's longest-living peoples. They grow well in cold climates like the Utah Wasatch Mountains, where I live.

3½ cups water/ice

1 cup dried (or fresh) goji berries—if fresh, decrease water by ½ cup

3 large collard leaves, including stems

5 small kale sprigs, including stems

Spinach, added until mixture reaches 6-cup line

⅓ cup raw, organic agave

1 banana, frozen in chunks

1 cup frozen blackberries

12 large frozen strawberries

3 apples or oranges

Soak goji berries in the water for the smoothie 30–60 minutes in advance. Then add all greens and blend until smooth. Add agave and fruit and blend again until smooth. Serve immediately, or refrigerate for up to 24 hours in glass jars and shake well before serving.

Grapefruit Cilantro Booster

2¾ cups water/ice

2 cups cilantro

10 dates, pitted

Spinach, added until mixture reaches 6-cup line

½ tsp. ground cinnamon

1 large pink grapefruit, peeled

1 D'Anjou pear

2 bananas, frozen in chunks

¼ whole lime, unpeeled

2 cups frozen mixed berries

Blend first 4 ingredients until smooth. Add remaining ingredients and blend until smooth. Serve immediately, or refrigerate for up to 24 hours in glass jars and shake well before serving. (This recipe becomes stronger tasting if not consumed immediately.)

Green Chocolate Cooler

Rave taste-test reviews from my four kids, and higher in calories and protein than most green smoothie recipes—good for those involved in athletic training. This is bright green but chocolate flavored!

3 cups ice water

½ vanilla bean

2 large kale leaves

Red leaf lettuce, added until mixture reaches 6-cup line

¼ cup cacao nibs or powdered chocolate

2 Granny Smith apples

2 mangoes, peeled and pits removed

2 bananas, frozen in chunks

½ cup almond butter

½ cup raw, organic agave

Blend first 4 ingredients until smooth. Add remaining ingredients and blend until smooth. Serve immediately, or refrigerate for up to 24 hours and shake well before serving.

Kale Tangelo Tonic

2½ cups water

1 bunch curly kale

10-ounce bag baby spinach

5 tangelos or clementines

1 banana, frozen in chunks

3 cups frozen mixed berries

¼ whole lemon

¼ cup raw, organic agave

Blend first 3 ingredients well. Add remaining ingredients, purée until smooth, and serve immediately, or refrigerate for up to 24 hours in glass jars and shake well before serving.

Key Lime Broccosprout Blend

2¾ cups water/ice

4 key limes (whole)

1 cup broccoli sprouts (from health food store or sprout them yourself)

Spinach, added until mixture reaches 6-cup line

3 D'Anjou pears

2 bananas, frozen in chunks

2 cups frozen mixed berries

1 tsp. stevia

Blend first 4 ingredients until smooth. Add remaining ingredients and blend until smooth. Serve immediately, or refrigerate for up to 24 hours in glass jars and shake well before serving.

Kiwi Banana Krush

2¾ cups water/ice

6 medium chard leaves

Spinach, added until mixture reaches 6-cup line

6 kiwis, peeled

1 banana, frozen in chunks

2 pears

3 cups frozen berries (until blender container is very full)

½ tsp. stevia or 2 Tbsp. raw, organic agave

Blend first 3 ingredients until smooth. Add fruit and stevia/agave and blend until smooth. Serve immediately for best results, or refrigerate up to 24 hours in glass jars and shake well before serving.

The Kumquat Question

2¾ cups water/ice

2 cups anise (fennel greens) (save the white fennel bulb for slicing into
    salads)

Spinach, added until mixture reaches 6-cup line

1 cup kumquats (including skin)

3 bananas, frozen in chunks

3 cups frozen mixed berries

¹/₃ cup raw, organic agave

Blend first 3 ingredients until smooth, then add remaining ingredients and
blend again until smooth. Serve immediately, or refrigerate for up to 24 hours in
glass jars and shake well before serving.

Late-Summer Apricot Watercress Divine

2¾ cups water/ice

1 bunch watercress

3 leaves kale (any kind)

Spring greens, added until mixture reaches 6-cup line

¼ lime

5–6 ripe apricots (optionally frozen in chunks)

2 ripe peaches (optionally frozen in chunks)

1 banana, frozen in chunks

1 cup blueberries

Blend first 5 ingredients until smooth, add fruit and blend again until
smooth. Serve immediately, or refrigerate for up to 24 hours in glass jars and
shake well before serving.

Latin Green Smoothie

3 cups water

½ bunch cilantro

2 inches fresh ginger, peeled

½ tsp. cayenne pepper

¼ cup raw, organic agave

Spinach and/or collards, added until mixture reaches 6-cup line

2 star fruit, coarsely chopped

½ lime, washed and quartered (including peel)

2 bananas, frozen in chunks

2 pears or apples

2 cups frozen mixed berries

Blend first 6 ingredients until smooth. Add remaining ingredients and blend until smooth. Serve immediately, or refrigerate for up to 24 hours in glass jars and shake well before serving.

Mango Meltaway

2¾ cups water/ice

2 stalks celery, chopped in fourths

Spinach, added until mixture reaches 6-cup line

½ cup cashews

½ tsp. vanilla

½ tsp. stevia

2 large mangoes, peeled and cut away from the pit

2 bananas, frozen in chunks

2 cups frozen blueberries

½ cup plain, nonfat yogurt or kefir

Blend first 4 ingredients until smooth, then add remaining ingredients and blend again until very smooth. Serve immediately for best results, or refrigerate up to 24 hours in glass jars and shake well before serving.

Melon-Seed Melange

It looks very green, but it's tasty! These ingredients are best when they're available in the very late summer or early fall.

¼ cup raw, organic agave

2 cups water

2 cups green cabbage

1 cup chopped parsley

Spinach, added until mixture reaches 6-cup line

4 cups cantaloupe, including all the seeds, etc., in the center (cut off peel)

2 bananas, frozen in chunks

12 medium to large frozen strawberries

Blend first 5 ingredients until very smooth. Add remaining ingredients and blend again until smooth. Serve immediately, or refrigerate for up to 24 hours in glass jars and shake well before serving.

Mixed Green Maca Madness

3 cups water/ice

Mixed spring greens, added to mixture up to 4-cup line

Spinach, added until mixture reaches 6-cup line

¼ cup maca root powder

½ tsp. lemon-flavored liquid stevia

2 cups pineapple

2 bananas, frozen in chunks

4 cups frozen berries

Blend first 3 ingredients until smooth. Add remaining ingredients and blend until smooth. Serve immediately for best results, or refrigerate up to 24 hours in glass jars and shake well before serving.

Mustard Greens Mambo

2¾ cups water/ice

2 large leaves (and stems) mustard greens, coarsely chopped

4 cups romaine, coarsely chopped

Spinach, added until mixture reaches 6-cup line

²/₃ tsp. powdered stevia

2 bananas, frozen in chunks

16 ounces frozen blackberries

1 small papaya, peeled (include the seeds in the smoothie)

2 apples, pears, or oranges

Blend first 4 ingredients until smooth, then add remaining ingredients and blend again until smooth. Serve immediately, or refrigerate for up to 24 hours in glass jars and shake well before serving.

One Really Grape Smoothie

2¾ cups water/ice

4 large handfuls mixed salad greens (such as sold in a tub at Costco)

Chard leaves (and stems), added until mixture reaches 6-cup line

1 banana, frozen in chunks

3 cups frozen mixed berries

2 cups seedless grapes (any kind)

2 Gala or Braeburn apples (add until blender container is very full)

¼ cup raw, organic agave

Blend first 3 ingredients until smooth. Add fruit and agave and blend until smooth. Serve immediately or refrigerate for up to 24 hours in glass jars and shake well before serving.

Pear Date Purée

2¾ cups water/ice

4 cups rainbow chard

Spinach, added until mixture reaches 6-cup line

¼ whole lemon

1 inch fresh ginger, peeled

6 large dates, or ⅓ cup chopped dates (rinsed)

3 large D'Anjou pears

3 cups frozen mixed berries

If possible, soak dates in water for 30 minutes. Blend first 6 ingredients until smooth. Add pears and berries and blend again until smooth. Serve immediately for best results, or refrigerate up to 24 hours in glass jars and shake well before serving.

Pollen Persimmon Potpourri

Bee pollen is famous for its aphrodisiac qualities as well as its ability to enhance your energy and many other health benefits. Raw local honey may help eliminate or reduce seasonal allergies.

2¾ cups water/ice

2 Tbsp. bee pollen

2 Tbsp. raw honey

½ tsp. cinnamon

¼ tsp. nutmeg

Spinach, added until mixture reaches 6-cup line

2 cups persimmons, chopped

1 banana, frozen in chunks

2 sweet apples, like Red or Golden Delicious

2 cups frozen blackberries

Blend first 6 ingredients until smooth. Add remaining ingredients and blend until smooth. Serve immediately, or refrigerate for up to 24 hours and shake well before serving.

Pomegranate Potion

Pomegranate juice has been an expensive "fad" health food for the past several years, as it's unusually high in polyphenols, tannins, and anthocyanins; the juice is higher in antioxidants than even green tea. Some studies documented decreases in blood pressure and cholesterol for those drinking the juice daily for a year. I'd still rather see you eat the whole food than a juice with a concentration of high sugars. You'll have lots of fiber from the pomegranate seeds, if not the concentration of nutrients that are not combinations found in nature anyway. Just buy a pomegranate when they're in season, peel away the red outer peel, break open the parts inside, and pop the ruby-like seeds out to eat. Children love the "treasure hunt" of removing the beautiful, juicy seeds in a pomegranate.

2¾ cups water/ice

5 large curly kale leaves

Spinach, added until mixture reaches 6-cup line

¼ cup raw, organic agave

4 tangerines or 2 oranges

1 banana, frozen in chunks

Seeds of 1 large pomegranate (1 cup or more)

2–3 Granny Smith apples

2 cups mixed frozen berries

Blend first 3 ingredients until smooth, then add remaining ingredients and blend again until smooth. Serve immediately, or refrigerate for up to 24 hours in glass jars and shake well before serving.

Rad Raspberry Radicchio

3 cups water/ice

2 large handfuls radicchio or red/purple cabbage

Spinach, added until mixture reaches 6-cup line

¼ cup raw, organic agave

2 cups frozen berries of any kind

3 tart-sweet (pink) apples, like Fuji or Jonathan

2 bananas, frozen in chunks

Blend first 3 ingredients until smooth. Add agave and fruit and blend until smooth. Serve immediately for best results, or refrigerate up to 24 hours in glass jars and shake well before serving.

Red Leaf Rocks

1 cup ice

1¾ cups water

1 head red leaf lettuce, washed

Collards, added until mixture reaches 6-cup line

½ lime (or 1–2 key limes), unpeeled

1 avocado, peeled and pit removed

2 Granny Smith (green) apples

1 banana, frozen in chunks

4 cups frozen mixed berries

½ tsp. stevia

Blend first 4 ingredients until smooth. Add fruit and stevia and blend until smooth. Serve immediately for best results, or refrigerate up to 24 hours in glass jars and shake well before serving.

Red Pepper Mint Julep

2¾ cups water

1 red bell pepper

1 large stalk celery

¼ whole lemon (including peel)

1 handful fresh mint leaves

Spinach, added until mixture reaches 6-cup line

½ tsp. stevia

1 Tbsp. bee pollen

2 apples

2 cups frozen mixed berries

4 cups frozen mixed fruit

1 banana, frozen in chunks

Blend first 6 ingredients until smooth. Add remaining ingredients and blend until smooth. Serve immediately, or refrigerate for up to 24 hours and shake well before serving.

Red Robyn Smoothie

2¾ cups water/ice

4 cups beet greens, coarsely chopped

Spinach, added until mixture reaches 6-cup line

½ tsp. stevia

12-ounce bag frozen pitted cherries

2 bananas, frozen in chunks

12 apricots, pitted

Blend first 3 ingredients until smooth. Add remaining ingredients and blend until smooth. Serve immediately or refrigerate for up to 24 hours in glass jars and shake well before serving.

Romaine Rounder

2¾ cups water/ice

2 stalks celery

1 carrot

Romaine lettuce, added until mixture reaches 6-cup line

½ tsp. stevia

1 ripe Bosc pear

8 apricots (preferably halved and frozen) or 4 peaches

2 bananas, frozen in chunks

2 cups frozen mixed berries

Blend first 4 ingredients until smooth. Add stevia and fruit and blend until smooth. Serve immediately for best results, or refrigerate up to 24 hours in glass jars and shake well before serving.

Savory Sweet-Hot Smoothie

2¾ cups water/ice

4 radishes and tops, washed well

3 ounces pea greens

Spinach, added until mixture reaches 6-cup line

¼ cup chopped dates

½ tsp. cayenne pepper

2 cups pineapple, preferably frozen in chunks

3 cups frozen berries

3 bananas, frozen in chunks

Blend first 4 ingredients until smooth. Add remaining ingredients and blend until smooth. Serve immediately for best nutrition (sprouts oxidize quickly), or refrigerate up to 24 hours in glass jars and shake well before serving.

Smooth Sunflowers

2¾ cups water/ice

2 ounces sprouted sunflower greens (grow your own or purchase at health
food store)

Spinach, added until mixture reaches 6-cup line

¼ whole lemon

I large Gala or Jonathan apple

2 bananas, frozen in chunks

2 small pears

2 cups frozen berries (or more, to fill container completely)

Blend first 3 ingredients until smooth. Add remaining ingredients and blend
until smooth. Serve immediately, or refrigerate for up to 24 hours in glass jars
and shake well before serving.

Sodium Dandelion Blast

Don't get sodium, the natural element and critical tissue binder, mixed up with
sodium chloride, the table salt. The former is highly necessary in your diet while
the latter should be avoided. Celery is an outstanding contributor of sodium and
is high on the maximum-nutrients-for-the-calorie scale, since you expend more
calories eating celery than you get from it!

2¾ cups water

2 large stalks celery

¼ whole lemon

2 inches fresh ginger, peeled

4 cups dandelion greens

Spinach, added and blended up to 6-cup line

2 oranges

2 bananas, frozen in chunks

Frozen berries added and blended until container is very full

Blend first 6 ingredients until smooth. Add fruit and blend until smooth.
Serve immediately, or refrigerate for up to 24 hours in glass jars and shake well
before serving.

South Pacific Green Smoothie

2¾ cups young Thai coconut liquid (or water)

4–6 large dates

Your favorite greens, added until mixture reaches 6-cup line

3 cups chopped fresh pineapple

1 cup young Thai coconut flesh

2 cups guanabana fruit or pulp (if you can find it, imported—if not, use any
    other fruit, like dark berries, if you don't want your smoothie to be
    bright green)

3 bananas, frozen in chunks

Blend first 3 ingredients until smooth. Add remaining ingredients and blend
again until smooth. Serve immediately for best nutrition, or store for up to 24
hours in glass jars in the fridge, shaking well before serving.

Southern Turnip-Collard Watermelon Cooler

These are popular ingredients in the South but can be found elsewhere, as well,
in the summer.

1 cup water

4 cups watermelon chunks

4 turnip green leaves (and stems), coarsely chopped

4 large collard leaves (and stems), coarsely chopped

¼ cup raw, organic agave

2 pears (or apples, oranges, etc.)

12 ounces frozen raspberries

2 bananas

Blend all ingredients together until very smooth. Serve immediately, or
refrigerate for up to 24 hours in glass jars and shake well before serving.

Sweet Beet Slam

3 cups water/ice

I large English cucumber (no need to peel it)

I large carrot

Beet greens, added until mixture reaches 6-cup line

½ tsp. cinnamon

⅓ cup agave

2 large, ripe pears (added till container is very full)

3 cups frozen mixed berries

I banana, frozen in chunks

Blend first 4 ingredients until smooth. Add remaining ingredients and blend until smooth. Serve immediately, or refrigerate for up to 24 hours in glass jars and shake well before serving.

Tomato Tonic

2 cups water/ice

I large English cucumber, washed and chopped into 2-inch pieces

I stalk celery, quartered

I large carrot, quartered

3 large, ripe Roma tomatoes

I large handful spinach

2 cloves fresh garlic

Pinch sea salt

Freshly ground pepper to taste

Tabasco or hot sauce to taste

Blend all ingredients until very smooth. Serve immediately.

Watercress Avocado Dream

2¾ cups water/ice

1 inch fresh ginger, peeled

¼ cup raw, organic agave

1 bunch watercress

2 stalks celery

1 ripe avocado

Spinach, added until mixture reaches 6-cup line

2 pears

2 bananas, frozen in chunks

Frozen mixed berries, added until container is very full

Blend first 7 ingredients in the order and quantities given. When mixture is very smooth, serve immediately, or refrigerate for up to 24 hours in glass jars and shake well before serving.

Appendix

Frequently Asked Questions: Dear GreenSmoothieGirl

Here are detailed answers to the frequently asked questions I get at GreenSmoothieGirl.com.

What should I store my green smoothie in to take to work or school? I have read about chemicals from synthetics like plastic leaching into liquids.

A government study by the nonprofit Environmental Working Group (EWG) in Washington, D.C., recently uncovered a surprising (and unnerving) finding. The plastic lining used by manufacturers of metal food cans have more bisphenol-A (BPA) than plastic containers do. BPA is an endocrine-disrupting chemical linked by research to breast and prostate cancer, diabetes, and neurological problems for babies exposed in utero, among other things. Cans that test at the highest BPA levels are chicken soup, infant formula, and canned pasta. And, the FDA says the average American eats about 17 percent canned foods. The longer a can sits on the shelf, the more leaching occurs in the food. And when a container is heated, more chemical is released into the food as well.

What can we do about this?

I believe that eventually BPA will be removed from cans. But, in the meantime, the first tip is that Eden Foods, a maker of organic items found mostly in health food stores, has BPA-free cans, if you can afford a pricier product.

Second, we can make more of our own food (like soups and beans) and keep canned food around only for food storage and emergencies. Cook the beans you use a lot and freeze them in two-cup amounts for later use. Some foods you buy in cans can be purchased in glass jars (spaghetti sauce, for instance).

Third, store your green smoothies in glass pint or quart jars. I've always done this. The downside is that if you drop it, glass shatters. So take it to work in a plastic bag, just in case it spills or breaks in transit, to protect the inside of your bag or briefcase or lunch cooler. Glass jars are admittedly not as convenient as some drink containers for taking in the car and putting in the car's drink holder. You can obtain stainless steel containers, too. With either of those options, you'll have no chemicals leaching into your food. Keep in mind that the best way to keep your body removing toxins like BPA from sources we just can't control is . . . to drink green smoothies! The insoluble plant fiber in greens mops up several times its own weight in toxins and removes them from the body.

Fourth, you can google "BPA free" and buy baby bottles and other items free of toxic synthetics.

A popular email has circulated about how a Johns Hopkins newsletter stated that Sheryl Crow's breast cancer was caused by dioxins leaching into the bottled water she drank.

Sheryl Crow doesn't know what caused her breast cancer any more than anyone else can isolate one factor like that (out of so many in our daily environment). Watchdog sites like truthorfiction.com and snopes.com were quick to repudiate the story. This should not, however, be taken as evidence that plastics are perfectly safe.

While this email has no accuracy, and highly dangerous dioxins do not leach from plastic into water, other toxic chemicals like phthalates do. Avoid bottled drinking water, which often contains more chemicals in the water than tap water does. Bottled water may be convenient, but rubbing a few brain cells together to fill our own water container not only saves us from drinking chemicals, it also decreases the impact on the environment. Currently well over one million drinking water bottles *daily* are filling up our garbage piles. My town of 10,000 people ships its garbage to a town two hours south, because our own landfills are full. One of the biggest-impact and lowest-sacrifice things we can do to ameliorate that situation is to swear off bottled water.

How long can I keep green smoothies in the fridge? Will they lose all their nutrients if I don't drink them right away?

Green smoothies are best when consumed immediately after blending them. Raw plant foods do oxidize rather quickly when the cells walls are broken down through blending and then exposed to air. However, fiber remains intact, the taste is still good, and the vast majority of nutrients are intact for about 24 hours after blending. I do occasionally drink green smoothies up to 48 hours later, but any longer than that, you're not going to like the taste. Always cover your green smoothies with a tight lid to minimize oxidation and avoid absorbing other smells/flavors from the refrigerator.

I just use mostly spinach in my smoothies. Do I have to use a lot of other greens if my family just likes spinach and not other greens?

I use spinach in almost every smoothie I make because it's abundantly and inexpensively available, mild in flavor, and smooth when blended, making concoctions even very young children will drink. However, the biggest variety possible of greens is best because of the wide variability in nutrients that you need for hundreds of physical functions. Even if spinach is your primary ingredient, branch out to add celery, kale, collards, and chard, at least. Celery is high in the fairly rare mineral sodium, kale has tremendous insoluble fiber—you get the idea. When you're a seasoned green smoothie pro, add smaller amounts of savory greens like mustard, dandelion, turnip greens, or arugula.

Can you overdose on spinach? Some people say there are compounds in spinach that can cause health problems.

I've been eating several handfuls of spinach virtually every day for 15 years without any negative health effects. A recent theory and opinion is that some greens (especially spinach) are high in oxalates and should be avoided because oxalates may interfere with absorption of calcium from the body and can cause kidney stones or gallbladder problems. Another popular opinion is that cooking spinach renders the oxalates harmless.

In fact, peer-reviewed research reveals that the ability of oxalates to lower calcium absorption is small and does not outweigh the ability of those foods to contribute significant calcium to the diet, since spinach is rich in calcium. A few rare health conditions require oxalate restriction: absorptive hypercalciuria type II, enteric hyperoxaluria, and primary hyperoxaluria. These are *not* the more common condition wherein kidney stones are formed.

Despite opinion propagated mostly via the Internet, research is not clear that restricting foods such as spinach helps prevent stones in those who have previously had them. Many researchers believe that dietary restriction cannot reduce risk of stone formation. In fact, some foods that were assumed to increase stone formation because of oxalate content (like black tea) have appeared in more recent research to have a preventative effect.

Further, cooking has a small impact (10 percent or less) on the oxalate content of foods, with no statistically significant lowering of oxalates following blanching or boiling of greens. A recent study suggests that blending foods containing oxalates, like we do making green smoothies, neutralizes those mineral-binding oxalate compounds. The nutritional advantages, then, of eating raw greens continue to far outweigh any benefit of cooking them.

Two other classes of nutritional compounds, *purines* and *goitrogens*, are found in some leafy greens such as spinach. Eating "excessive" amounts of spinach or cruciferous vegetables (like broccoli) containing these compounds can be a problem for people who suffer with gout, kidney stones, or low thyroid hormone production. (Ironically, these are diseases that could possibly have been avoided with lifelong high greens and vegetable/fruit consumption.) These chemical compounds are also found in peanuts, strawberries, soy products, and other foods. Lightly steaming these foods may help. However, the literature seems to support the idea that a few weekly servings of these foods is good for almost everyone and does not constitute "excessive amounts."

What about E. Coli?

I'm often asked about whether I'm scared of spinach after the E. Coli scare in 2006. I'm not afraid of it at all. A ten-year study done by Centers for Disease Control proved that eating raw plant foods is the safest strategy, because less than one-tenth of 1 percent of food-borne diseases are caused by raw plant foods. All the others are caused by animal and/or cooked foods.

In fact, I'm pretty sure my kids and I ate some E. Coli-tainted spinach, a couple of days in a row, during the outbreak in 2006. I barely noticed it. People with healthy gastrointestinal tracts who eat excellent nutrition every day are not generally the ones who succumb to parasites and intestinal bacteria. If you eat plenty of raw, nutrition-dense plant fiber and stay away from foods that compromise your immune function, after a possible initial cleansing period, you'll likely find that you go through the winter without falling prey to the viruses that are felling everyone around you.

You can't eliminate all risk of food-borne illness. But, as a strategy, eliminating greens is the least-wise strategy toward that end I can think of. Keeping your body clean with lots of organic, raw plant food is simply the best strategy I know of to minimize disease risk of all kinds—degenerative diseases, food-borne illnesses, and viral and bacterial infections.

Can I freeze green smoothies?

Yes. One GreenSmoothieGirl.com reader said she froze a quantity of green smoothies in pint jars for a road trip she took. She then put them all in a cooler covered with ice, and took one out a few hours before she wanted to drink it, twice a day. This way she had excellent nutrition throughout her weeklong trip, without having to take her high-power blender along and make a mess in a hotel room. (That is something I've done on a regular basis, though her idea is better.)

Freezing does not preserve 100 percent of nutrients, but it's the best method of preservation, and enzymes do survive freezing. Produce stored in a small freezer should be used within a few weeks, ideally, for minimal nutrient loss, or within a few months in a larger deep freeze.

Isn't it bad to combine fruits and vegetables?

A very few in the field of nutrition forward theories about "food combining"—that certain foods shouldn't be combined or the gut has difficulty digesting. Animal proteins and fruits, for instance, according to some, shouldn't be consumed together, since fruit is digested in 20–45 minutes, and protein takes hours.

Some say that starchy vegetables and fruits shouldn't go together, either. I can't find any true evidence that this will cause you problems, but if you personally find that this food combination causes you problems (potatoes with fruits, for instance), then don't put carrots in your green smoothies. If there were a valid food combination to avoid, I believe it would be animal flesh and fruit.

However, greens belong in their own class. They're not vegetables—they're greens. They're excellent combined with fruit, by anyone's standards.

Take "food combining" theory with a grain of salt, because plenty of experts feel that worrying about food combinations is pointless and your body has the capacity to handle the various combinations. I'm skeptical of anything that makes our ability to nourish ourselves "rocket science" or a source of worry and stress. Are you eating all whole foods and avoiding meat, dairy, and processed foods? If not, that's a more pressing concern than worrying about whether you ate carrots and peaches together in the same meal.

How much should an adult drink, and how much should I give my child?

I recommend that an adult make a goal to drink one quart daily. An ambitious goal for a child is to have him or her drink a pint daily. That's 15 servings of greens and fruit for you and 7.5 adult servings for your child, according to the FDA.

If a pint daily is too much for your child, in the beginning, start with less and work your way toward that as a goal. You might achieve a pint by having him drink half at lunch and half with his afternoon snack. My kids know their green smoothie is the first thing they drink, and they're allowed to have whatever else only when it's gone. See "Tips for Helping Kids Go Green" (page 68) in this book.

Sometimes when I feel in need of detoxification or want to lose a couple of pounds, I eat a normal breakfast, and then drink a quart of green smoothie for lunch and another quart for dinner. Being a single mom now, I take advantage of periods when my children are at their father's to avoid food prep, except green smoothies in the blender, and I practically live on them. Doing this (drinking half a gallon a day) will accelerate cleansing in the body; it could cause diarrhea and temporarily overwhelm some of your organs of elimination if you haven't been on a mostly whole-food, plant-based diet for quite a while.

For about a year, a woman who weighed well over 500 pounds undertook a "green smoothie experiment" and blogged about her five months of eating nothing but green smoothies. She lost over 100 pounds during that period of time and documented many positive health changes. She also suffered some challenging detox symptoms in the beginning, of course. You may still be able to find her blog by googling "green smoothie experiment."

Do I have to blend the greens first, and then the fruit?

No. I just do it that way to make sure that no chunks of greens remain (which my kids don't appreciate), and to obtain plenty of liquid before adding frozen fruit, just to make the blending process as easy as possible.

How can enzymes and eating raw food be so important
when stomach acid would kill any enzymes that came with the
food anyway?

Good question. Some people think that the low pH of the stomach stops salivary and any other food or supplemental enzymes from working. A number of experiments Dr. Edward Howell writes about show that this is not so. Some enzymes are shown to work actively at two different pH ranges. Another study shows that salivary and supplemental enzymes were re-activated in the alkaline duodenum and lower in the intestine after going through the stomach. Hydrochloric acid in the stomach is not as strong as once thought to be and neither when used in in vitro experiments (outside the body). A *Journal of Nutrition*–published study at Northwestern University showed 51 percent of amylase from malted barley was intact when passed into the intestine.

Enzymes manufactured by the pancreas of a person or animal are sensitive to pH because they aren't adapted to anything outside the restrictive confines of the body. But microbial-derived dietary supplement enzymes are very adaptive, since fungus grows in a variety of places and conditions. These enzymes survive the acidity of the lower stomach.

These plant-based sources are the digestive enzyme supplements I prefer.

As with so many other things in the human body, we've been provided with the ideal environment to digest food. Problems occur when we alter our food instead of giving our body the kind of nutrition we were designed to digest easily, that people used to eat for thousands of years.

Dr. Howell says that we're born with a finite ability to produce endogenous enzymes, and by middle age, most of that ability is gone. (And he said this 25 years ago, before the modern diet worsened. Some experts make even more dire projections, such as Westerners are burning out enzyme capacity by age 35.) The answer, of course, is to eat as much raw food as possible, and as little cooked or processed food, too.

Sometimes I feel nauseated when I drink green smoothies. What can I do?

Although it's a small minority of green smoothies drinkers who experience this, it's not entirely uncommon, especially if you drink your whole quart in one sitting. This should not be taken as a sign that your body doesn't use the nutrition in your blended drinks well, but, rather, you need to eat some other solid food along with your smoothie. Some of my readers report that if they eat some complex carbohydrates and/or good fats, they don't experience that symptom. Consider a handful of raw almonds, some brown rice prepared however you like it, an avocado (or homemade guacamole with sprouted-wheat tortilla chips), or a piece of whole-grain toast as accompaniments. (My friend Richard mashes an avocado, spreads it on wheat berry bread, drizzles it with honey, and calls it the best treat in the world.)

If you're trying to drink a quart daily, consider drinking a pint twice a day, instead, with other food. Your body will be able to use all that nutrition better anyway, in two sittings.

Also consider adding a chunk of fresh ginger to your smoothies; it's an excellent anti-nausea remedy and a power food for a variety of other reasons, as well.

This is kind of a personal (and slightly embarrassing) question here but I really need to ask it. Are green feces normal when drinking green smoothies? Is that a good or bad sign?

This is a big and important topic, involving a 100-foot-long tract plus a number of organs in your body most of us know little about. People in the Western world are shockingly uneducated on this topic because of the social taboo involved with talking about it. So, learn about it here in the safety of this book, where no one will know you're learning about feces.

Green bowel movements are completely normal (that's the plant fiber in all those greens you're eating)! Take a look at the horse poop you see along the road, if you live where you can see horses. It's indicative of what they eat (alfalfa, all plant foods). You can read about indigenous people who have no toilets and, therefore, "squat" outside. They don't worry about human waste removal like we do, because it's not toxic and disgusting, like it would be here in the U.S. The poop of indigenous people who eat mostly raw plant food looks like horse poop: lots of it, lots of fiber in it, greenish, with no odor. Brown feces are simply a result of bile pigments coming from the liver, also normal.

What you should be concerned about is dark, hard, smelly, putrefied poop—that's what most of America is experiencing. (And, that, I believe, is why we're so shamed about the topic of elimination—the feces of people eating the S.A.D. are,

in fact, disgusting!) That's what eating meat gets you: putrefied stool that takes days (or, with pork, even weeks) to digest.
Accumulation of decaying material in the digestive tract,
euphemistically known as constipation, is the single biggest
threat to our health, the "modern plague," according to Dr.
Bernard Jensen.

I helped run a babysitting co-op for ten years while my
children were small, and I was always horrified when I had to
change other babies' diapers—the smell was astonishing. I was
at a party where everyone watched and laughed as a toddler
was straining, his face beet red, trying to have a bowel movement in his diaper. This little boy was fed a steady diet of hot
dogs and potato chips, zero-fiber foods. I never once saw any
of my four children do that. Many parents have come to think
of that phenomenon as normal, but it's not: Straining at a
bowel movement is constipation, plain and simple.

People get painful hemorrhoids—bulging, inflamed veins
pop out of the anus instead of staying inside like they
should—when their colons are overtaxed with low-fiber foods
and they must exert lots of force to eliminate. That's just one
of the many side effects of eating a low-fiber diet.

Diverticulitis is a very dangerous disease caused by chronic constipation; pouches of the colon sag, lose nerve and muscle tone, and become breeding grounds for bacteria that eventually rot the colon. Meat is a major culprit, and constipation
is well catalogued as a common complaint in any honest
review of results of the Atkins Diet, since anyone on that diet
is excessively eating animal proteins.

But Dr. Bernard Jensen and his researchers, tracking
10,000 people's colon health over decades of his practice, constantly noted that those suffering from the worst colon prob-

lems ate lots of white bread, which functions like the gluey mess that it is, slowing and gumming up your digestive system. He said that anyone eating refined flour better be eating lots of vegetable roughage at the same time (and he recommends whole millet, rye, cornmeal, and rice, instead).

People who eat lots of plant food have soft but formed stool. People who have been eating an almost exclusively plant-based diet for a long time, and have been through all the "cleansing" so they're now rather clean, have—it sounds trite at best and ridiculous at worst, but it's a well-kept secret—poop that doesn't stink.

Ever since I started on green smoothies, I have flatulence! Help!

A healthy bowel produces minimal flatulence, none of it foul smelling or causing pressure, swelling, or pain. Gas is, as Dr. Bernard Jensen described it, "putrefactive fermentations" of undigested proteins. In other words, proteins sit in the gut and become hosts for undesirable bacteria.

The problem is, when converting people to a high-fiber, GreenSmoothieGirl diet, some people who didn't have gas before now do! If they drank Coke and ate donuts before, they had no flatulence, but then when they start green smoothies to begin their progression toward a whole-foods diet, they're gassy and miserable. They might even want to quit and go back to when they felt "better."

Dr. Jensen likened this to when you sweep a dirty basement: as you sweep it up, a lot of dust is kicked into the air. His research indicates, however, that people, even while experiencing gas problems, report softer stool and an easier time passing off the gas. It gradually lessens, he said, until it becomes minimal after about three months. (My own observations from working with people are that most people see this symptom disappear in weeks rather than months.) Be patient and don't quit good habits as you seek relief for intestinal gas and bloating.

As you get through that initial period, drink 1 ounce of water for every 2 pounds of body weight, which will help.

Green Smoothie Testimonials

By following Robyn's recommendation, which I could not believe at first but made a decision to try, I lost weight without trying, and my knees and shoulders stopped aching. My blood lipid profile has improved. My cholesterol level has gone from 201 down to 157. Yes, I said 157. My doctor had me go to a different lab to have the test confirmed.

My complexion and skin tone have improved as well. I also had a problem with dry skin. I used coconut oil as recommended by Robyn, and my rash on my ankles and chin cleared up completely. I had gone to the doctor and obtained two different medications and the only thing that did any good and, in fact, cleared it up was the coconut oil. Thank you.

—*Sandra T.; California*

I have medulary sponge kidney disease that causes me to make kidney stones. My urologist sees me every 6 months to keep an eye on things. I started drinking green smoothies about 5 weeks ago, having 2 a day most days. I lost 6 pounds in 3 weeks, and haven't gained it back. About 10 days ago I had an ultrasound of my kidneys and 5 days ago I had the usual blood work done. I recently noticed my face (I'm always complimented on my youthful appearance) glowing—and my husband obviously thought so because he reached out to stroke my cheek with the back of his hand. I asked if I had food on my face and he said no. Then he stroked my cheek again.

Back to today's checkup with my urologist. He was very pleased, saying, "You always have many kidney stones in both kidneys—usually the left has more than the right, but they both have multiple stones. Your scan shows *no* stones in the left, and a stone the size of a pin point in the right kidney." He had to rock the wand forward and back to find it! He said, "You've lost weight. You look great! Whatever you're doing, keep it up! I don't need to see you for a year."

Here's the kicker: In the past he asked me to stay away from "high-oxalate" foods such as kale and spinach since my kidney stones are calcium-oxalate stones. But what greens have I put in my green smoothies? Kale, spinach, and beet tops. And I'm better than I've been in *years and years* in terms of kidney health.

Go green smoothies!

—*Cindy*

I'm at my ideal weight (have never been anywhere near over-weight), and I run or lift weights six days a week, and eat a healthy diet. Imagine my shock when I went to a clinic and was told I was prediabetic, that it was just a matter of time before I had full-blown diabetes. I burst out laughing when the nurse practitioner told me her recommendation was to cut out sugar, since I eat so little of it already. Robyn taught me about green smoothies, and I began making them daily for my family, as well as teaching others about them. I just went back to the clinic after several months of my new green-smoothie habit, and they said all signs of the prediabetic condition were gone. The only thing I changed was adding green smoothies to my diet!

—*Laura B.; Utah*

Green smoothies saved me from facing yet another diet, thinking about hypnosis for weight loss, hating the way I looked, and everything else that comes along with being overweight. Green smoothies are my answer to staying away from the doctor. I no longer have cravings and feel satisfied for hours after drinking my awesome smoothies. My husband is loving them, too, and has lost 40 pounds. The children love green smoothies. I appreciate all the information Robyn has shared. Thank you so much, Robyn!

—*A. Fambrough*

The power of peer influence is impressive. I'd been drinking green smoothies regularly for several months, but had yet to convince my children to participate. One day I was looking at www.GreenSmoothieGirl.com and my children, ages 4–12, were looking over my shoulder. They saw a picture of Emma, flexing, with her green smoothie, and my daughter said, "Wow—she's buff!" That day they all had a small glass of green smoothie for the first time! I guess kids really will drink them.

—*Leslie S.; Utah*

Robyn first told me about green smoothies about a year and a half ago. I dabbled with making them at first, but once I figured out what recipes worked well for me, I became hooked! I make a big green smoothie every morning for breakfast, and I finally don't have a late-morning energy crash like I used to. As a busy college student, it's become the perfect fast food— how else am I going to get all these great veggies into my diet before noon? I find the smoothies refreshing and surprisingly filling (especially if I add an avocado), and if I eat something else for breakfast one morning, I always end up making a green smoothie later in the day because I miss it! Both my mom and sister are hooked now, too, and make them every morning for breakfast.

—*Laura T.; California*

Is it possible to be addicted to green smoothies? Ever since you first introduced me to green drinks years ago, I've dabbled here and there with them. I decided to make green smoothies my daily morning meal—there isn't a quicker, more nutritious breakfast to be had! I've introduced green smoothies to my friends at the office, and even whip up an extra drink for one of my coworkers, who now says she can't wait for Monday mornings to come so she can have a smoothie for breakfast! I love the way I feel since incorporating green smoothies into my daily diet! I have energy for the entire morning; I do not crave sugar nearly as much. I can definitely say without doubt that green smoothies have made a difference; I just feel healthy!

This past week I made a green smoothie for a little nephew of mine who has never, ever eaten a vegetable in his life. Ever. My sister was very skeptical that he would even try it, let alone like it. Not only did he like it, he asked for more. My sister was blown away, and soooo happy to know that there was a way to get her little guy to get so much more nutrition into his diet. Oh, my sister loved it, too!

Thanks, Robyn, for introducing us slowly but surely to green-drink heaven! If I miss a day of green smoothies, I miss them, *crave* them, even. I've become a true addict.

—*Sheri H.; Utah*

Our family has been drinking green smoothies for the last 3 months and I feel it has improved our overall health. It has completely taken away the guilt in regards to my children's diet. I no longer have to worry about if they've gotten enough fruits and vegetables. I give them healthy snacks to eat, but on crazy, hectic days even if they have not had one other fruit or vegetable, I don't worry because they've had their green smoothie! I have a 5- and 3-year-old and worried if they would drink it. My 5-year-old loves it and many days asks for seconds and my 3-year-old occasionally has to be reminded to drink his smoothie, but it was a lot easier to get them to drink it than I imagined it would be—I add quite a few frozen strawberries to our smoothies and they really like it.

My husband just had a bone marrow transplant and we are very conscious that good nutrition is a key element in his recovery. One of the benefits I have experienced is I feel it has helped me keep up my milk supply for my newborn. I have had milk supply issues in the past and I am nursing my third baby longer than I was able to nurse my other two children. I feel green smoothies have played a part in my ability to do this. Green smoothies are a great way to make sure your family is getting all the fruits and vegetables they need to be as healthy as they possibly can be!

—*Quinn S.; North Carolina*

The green smoothie idea has worked well for me whereas juicing did not. Anyone who has juiced knows the time commitment it takes for juicing and cleanup, as well as the volume of veggies it takes to make just 2–3 eight-ounce juice drinks per day. When I read about green smoothies, it was immediately appealing to me. I bought a Blendtec right away. In only 14 months of use, the counter on my machine is already over 1,600!

I average 5 out of 7 days for making smoothies for me and my husband, who will drink one anytime it's available in the fridge. One benefit of green smoothies is that they're helping me to be more alkaline.

—*Linda C.*

When Robyn introduced me to green smoothies, I was intrigued by the idea of drinking my greens. I eat lots of fruits and vegetables in my diet, but I was looking for an easy way to double my fiber. I love green smoothies. I don't just drink a glass or two, but three or four, and then whatever is left over after my children drink theirs. I feel better. I feel thinner. But, by measurable standards—the scale, the tape measure—I am thinner.

The combination of green smoothies and lots of water promote weight loss in me. Feeling better about myself, I have a brighter outlook on life, naturally, but I simply have more energy to meet the demands and challenges of my busy days.

—Jill W.; Utah

My family—including my picky 2-year-old—really enjoys green smoothies. We like the fact that we're taking a significant step toward better health, and we've had far fewer illnesses since incorporating them into our diet. We've also made them for visiting family and friends, and they're all pleasantly surprised at how good they taste.

—Kari W.; Utah

I'm 44 years old. I've always had very regular menstrual cycles. For about one year prior to drinking green smoothies, my menstrual cycles had become very irregular. After about two months of green smoothies, I returned to a very regular cycle of 20–30 days and my periods are just like they were in my 20s and 30s. I've been drinking my quart of green smoothie per day for six months now and my cycles are consistently regular.

—Kathy M.

I love green smoothies! I drink them every morning, and I was so surprised how great they make me feel! I have lost weight, have lots of energy, feel healthier than ever, and feel like my immune system is even stronger than it was.

Drinking green smoothies also influenced all of my eating and cooking decisions, and allowed me to lose weight safely. When we travel, I am always carrying my blender with me so I can have green smoothies anywhere I go!

My 20-month-old daughter also loves them. I am sure that green smoothies are the best way to get babies and toddlers to get their greens. She gets so excited when I get out the blender and she always wants more! Thank you, green smoothies, and thank you to my friend, Tara, for introducing them to me!

—*Kathryn Rose*

I drink a quart of an all-vegetable green smoothie every day. I have more energy, sleep better, wake up ready for the day, and generally feel much better. I believe it's because of the green smoothie and a whole-foods diet, mostly raw. I have cut out all processed foods, sugar, and caffeine, and I feel great! Thanks for your website; it's very informative and inspiring!

—*Carol J.*

After a few weeks of drinking green smoothies via a wimpy blender, we were hooked and made our best nutritional investment to date—Blendtec. Our green smoothies have become greener and we have been known to eat 3–4 bunches of greens and 1 pound of baby spinach in a week between two adults and two toddlers.

I sometimes find myself looking around at all the green plants and wonder, "What would that taste like?" I was skeptical at first, but my then-barely-two-year-old and three-year-old both enjoyed the green smoothies as well. They were converted before my husband!

Summer proves to be an easier time to drink them due to the warmer weather. However, we still maintain regular GS drinking throughout all the seasons. I do not have to force them on my toddlers; rather, they will request them and are especially excited to help put all the ingredients into the blender.

GS have helped control my sugar cravings, eliminated Irritable Bowel Syndrome, and boosted my energy. My kids have regular bowel movements that do not have the stench as pre-GS days.

It is best to start children early on GS as it will develop their palate toward *real*, nutritionally sound foods.

—*Laura M. and family*

I wish I started drinking green smoothies earlier in life! I cannot believe how much energy I have just from this one simple dietary change! My digestion issues vanished in one week and my skin looks amazing. I feel really healthy and cannot say enough about how much more energy I have.

—*Anon.*

I crave green smoothies. They satisfy my hunger. I am a teacher; therefore, I am surrounded by germs and viruses. Since I have been on green smoothies for about six months, I have not been sick. I am convinced the phytonutrients in my breakfast and lunch smoothie are what have kept me in good health.

—*Chris B.*

I am so in love with green smoothies! I am a 31-year-old mother of four children. I am very into fitness and weight lifting to build muscle in my body. I started green smoothies just after I had been referred to GreenSmoothieGirl.com by my zoning lady for chronic headaches and muscle tension in my neck that would not go away. Soon after I started drinking green smoothies daily, the headaches and muscle tension left! I have not had the problem since.

I drink green smoothies for breakfast along with a protein shake every morning, and also for my snacks during the day. I make a full pitcher of green smoothie every 2–3 days and keep it in my fridge. It is quick and easy and very healthy! It keeps me on track for my ideal weight goals! I have converted many friends and family to green smoothies! I recommend them to everyone I meet! When someone asks me what I am doing to look so good, I just give them my personal green smoothie recipe and some fitness tips!

I would like to thank Robyn for this *awesome* idea and for taking the steps to get the information on her website to help others who so desperately need a nutritious lifestyle!

—*LaDawn Doxey; Syracuse, Utah*

Feel better, have decreased the amount of sugar in the diet due to the smoothies. Like the increase in green veggies. Hate the taste of wheatgrass. Like this manner of getting chlorophyll better.

—*Anon.*

I would like to convert everybody. There are many benefits. You will experience increased energy. You will need less sleep and your cravings for sweets will decrease down to nothing. You will lose weight, your blood pressure will come down. You will feel 21 again.

I actually really look forward to the first smoothie in the a.m. It is easy, and if you give it a chance, you will love it, too. The first smoothie I made I used half a banana and it tasted great, but I did not want to use it on a daily basis. So, I did not make any smoothies for one month. I decided to go back and try again, this time with half an apple for 32 ounces. That hooked me!

Green smoothies taste so fresh. I make 64 ounces in the a.m. I use 32 ounces in the morning and save the next 32 ounces for noon meal. You can take it with you to work. It travels well and it is so easy, I just make mine fresh every day.

The GreenSmoothieGirl website is extremely informative with all the information for making the green smoothie. I vary the greens (very important), but my base is apple, celery, parsley (all organic, of course). Then, on various days, I use two of the following: any of the types of kale, Swiss chard, mustard greens, collard greens, dandelion, arugula, or anything else that looks fresh.

Put the soft washed leafy greens in the bottom of the blender and top it with the harder washed vegetables. Add the filtered water, and start blending. If it is too thick, add more water and blend again. I sip it (as a good portion of digestion occurs in the mouth). And I get to enjoy this every morning.

Now, to keep the greens extra fresh, here is what I do. I place each type of green unwashed in a Mason jar one-quarter filled with water. I top it with one of those green bags and twist the green bag at the bottom around with my fingers, so it is fairly secure around the Mason jar. Greens keep great, and I never throw out anything, seriously. Keeping green onions like this is wonderful, the greens love it. Wishing my best to everyone who has a desire for great health and is willing to give a green smoothie a fair shot.

—*Lorraine L.; Naples, Florida*

What can we say! My husband, our 15-month-old baby, and I are hooked! There is no such thing as the 3 o'clock sleepiness anymore. We have so much more energy. Our daughter loves the smoothies. She even has a smoothie dance she does when she wants some. With her on the green smoothies, I do not worry so much about if she is getting proper nutrition. I just know she is. With the addition of flaxseed or chia, I also know she is getting the good fats she needs for brain development. I am so glad I stumbled onto your site, Robyn. This has changed our lives.

—*Shelly N.*

This is the healthful "fast food!" My health has changed for the better! I now have a desire to do, and to live! Thanks to green smoothies!

—*Dallas J.*

I tried the green smoothie after juicing for several years. Juicing was expensive and demanded a lot of time and work extracting the juice from the fiber and cleaning the juicer. Blended raw foods made a lot of sense and I did not need to be converted to the idea.

When I began drinking the green smoothie I weighed 285 pounds. One year later I weigh 240 pounds. Daily workouts have contributed as much to my weight loss as any other factor. However, the benefits of the green smoothie as I experienced them are as follows:

1. Drinking the green smoothie changed my bowel movement habits, which are now frequent (2–3 times a day) and regular.

2. The green smoothie is my pre-workout, first-thing-in-the-morning food. I have been surprised at the energy it sustains throughout my workout.

3. The green smoothie fills me up without slowing me down. It satisfies my hunger and cravings till early in the

afternoon. It has curbed my overall appetite, thus decreasing the overall calories I consume in a day.

4. I find that the green smoothie helps my digestion, especially with the foods that do not digest well. I eat a lot of lean meat and I feel the organic raw food in my gut facilitates digestion and elimination of meat.

5. Beginning my day with green smoothie drinks and working out provides me the momentum, nutrition, and motivation to eat a strict lean diet throughout the rest of the day.

The green smoothie has lived up to the expectations I had. Several of the above benefits caught me totally by surprise. I have been drinking green smoothies every morning for the past year. They have served me well. Now that I have lost the weight I needed, I have significantly increased my strength and energy. My new goals are not to lose any more weight but to increase my overall lean muscle mass. My idea is to begin drinking green smoothies twice a day rather than just once in the morning.

—*Gregg L.*

I started drinking green smoothies and doing about 80–95 percent raw to help improve my migraine headaches. I lost 51 pounds in six months and I feel great. I am 47 years old, and I teach at an alternative high school. It can be very stressful working with at-risk youth. I have seen my mood and attitude improve so much since I started adding green smoothies as my breakfast.

My favorite is 2 bananas, 1 large apple, 2 kale leaves, 6–8 dandelion greens, 2 large handfuls fresh spinach, some wheatgrass juice, 2 cups water, and 1 cup of ice. Blend and I have breakfast and my afternoon snack. This is great stuff and I will never go back to eating the way I used to with fast and processed foods.

—*Carol N.*

I have endometriosis and ovarian cysts and have suffered with cramping, heavy menstruation, and low back pain for 20-plus years. I have had numerous surgeries to help correct and alleviate the problem with no success. I finally reached the point that my doctors determined a hysterectomy would be my next surgery. I am in my early thirties and was not ready for that so I spent a lot of time researching nutritional options. I discovered green smoothies and they have helped tremendously (I have been drinking them for a year now).

My cycles have improved dramatically and the majority of the time I feel like a normal person. That has never been the case because of this constant pain that was always with me. Thanks for all of the info on your site. As I have changed my eating habits I have also discovered trigger foods that cause ovarian pain, spotting, and bleeding. I am grieving the loss of chocolate but the smoothies have almost taken any cravings for sweets away. Once again thanks so much for helping to change the quality of my life.

—*Becky Flannery; Sandy, Utah*

I started drinking green smoothies two months ago. I use a large amount of organic leafy produce and I use kombucha as the liquid, with a small amount of fruit or fruit juice. Then I follow it up with a handful of spirulina and chlorella tablets. This combination rocks.

—*Anon.*

Green smoothies have saved my life! I had been in a state of depression for the past 4 years. I was put on depression medicine but it never helped. I discovered green smoothies in December 2008 and decided to give it a try in January 2009. It has been two months since I started making a green smoothie every day and I feel *amazing, wonderful,* and *full of life.* I have not felt this good in a long time. I have had tons of energy; I can fall asleep faster at night and feel rested when I wake up; I don't feel the need to take daily naps; I have had less cravings for sweets and processed foods; my motivation is back; and I have lost 8 pounds in 2 months. Green smoothies are here to stay!

—*Alessa Brennan*

I love the green smoothies; they have made a world of difference in my life. I know I am a happier, healthier person because of them. I am so thankful for them; I love them so very much. They have given me so much drive. It is easier to drink your greens. I have been eating healthy greens for years. I like the kale in a smoothie rather than eating it daily as I have done. It is much easier to get down in a drinkable form. Thank you!

—*Lisa*

I have been drinking green smoothies for almost a year now. They are delicious and refreshing. I have had to travel during that time period which caused me to abandon my smoothie for 10 days and I have *really* felt the effects (fatigue). I will never stop drinking green smoothies!

—*Anon.*

I have been telling all my friends about the green smoothies and converted several of them to start drinking them on a daily basis. My friends are all West Coast dancers and energy is important for the 4–5 hours of dancing we do 2–3 nights weekly.

—*Anon.*

I have had an iron deficiency most of my life and the green smoothies have helped tremendously! I am losing less hair in the shower as a result. My daughters (age 6, 7, and 10) love the green smoothies! They even ask for them now and love watching me make them. It is so good to be able to give them a way to get good veggies in their diet without fighting with them. Thank you for changing our way of life.

—*JoAnn Y.; Denver, Colorado*

I have become so converted to green smoothies that I became concerned as to how to continue them in case of disaster or hard economic times when I might be unable to purchase fresh produce. So I started dehydrating the spinach, kale, and parsley I grew in my garden this year. I then powdered the dried leaves and use it during the winter to make my green smoothies.

For the juice base, I use frozen raw apple cider that my husband grinds fresh each fall with his leftover apples (he is a fruit farmer). It is now January and I use the following recipe for my super green smoothies:

I rehydrate in 1 cup hot water the following: 2 teaspoons powdered kale plus a half teaspoon powdered parsley or 2 1/2 teaspoons powdered spinach. Blend well and let sit for about 10 minutes, until cooled. Then add 3 cups apple juice (raw, unpasteurized), 2 frozen bananas, 1 1/2 tablespoons freshly ground flaxseed, and water and ice to the 7-cup mark and thoroughly blend. This is a great option when I cannot get to the grocery store.

—*Cindy P.; Alpine, Utah*

Green smoothies are now a daily part of my life! I have much more energy now and GS is a complete meal, more nutritious than eating out! I have been a vegetarian for 30 years and this has definitely improved my health! As a teacher (now retired)

and a lifeguard for the Kentucky State Park System for 32 summers, green smoothies help me to stay in great shape!
—*Steve House*

We love green smoothies at our house. I am a homeschooling mom of four children. Three of my children drink smoothies because they love them, and one child drinks her smoothies because it's a good health choice. I try to vary the ingredients here and there so that they don't get bored with them. We drink them first thing in the morning. I also have been known to feed them to neighbor children who then will ask to have more! Also, they are pretty tasty as popsicles: I am sure they lose some nutrition being frozen, but the kids love them!
—*Melanie H.*

My family and I have been drinking green smoothies for 8 months. It has been our addiction. If I miss a day, I feel it and crave it instead of cake. My kids who are 9 and 6 actually ask me for them, so they have some before school. I no longer have pre-hypertension and I have lost 25 pounds. My husband no longer has to take his cholesterol medication and has lost weight. My best friend now gives it to her whole family and staff every day. And another friend who just completed chemo will be starting also. Thank you!
—*Lisa James*

Even if I have not seen so much difference, I feel lucky to have been introduced to green smoothies, a very interesting way to eat more greens and fruits. Hope it will show results in a near future and keep disease at bay!

I now fix green smoothies for my entire family several times per week and our immune systems have been clearly better while doing this on a consistent basis.
—*Anon.*

I look forward every morning to drinking my green smoothie because I know that it is a delicious, healthy, and empowering way to start my day. I now have my husband converted and my college-age son who needs good nutrition because most of the other things he grabs during the day are fast, on-the-go foods. I feel full of raw goodness and do not need to eat anything else for most of the morning.

—*Ciel M.*

Green smoothies are easy and quick to do and keep me full and alert way past lunchtime. This past growing season I had access to lots and lots of lettuce. I would use between 2 and 3 cups in my smoothie along with other greens, but long after the other greens were gone there was still plenty of leaf lettuce in many colors and kinds. All of my greens came from my local farmers' market.

—*Anon.*

I wish my mother had fed me green smoothies from birth. If she had I would not have had all this pain and suffering I have been through. I understand nowadays that my body was only crying out for help from me. I only wish all people I know—soon— will come to understand this. Good health to all. Thanks!

—*Anon.*

I have enjoyed physical changes in my body. I have enjoyed some weight loss, great digestion, and increased desire to reduce cooked and processed foods. I have talked to others about using the green smoothies as a means to improve their overall health.

—*C. Brown*

I feel that prayer led me to your website, and looking at the other testimonials, this seems to be a common theme! What a blessing to have such information at my fingertips! I felt good about the smoothies, and they made obvious sense to me, so I decided to make them. Imagine my surprise, therefore, when suddenly all of my pregnancy fat from the last two kids melted away (I haven't worn this size jeans in 3 years) and I found myself struggling to get enough calories to nurse!

My husband has noticed a definite improvement in my attitude after I started a colon cleanse (smoothies clean out your liver, and everything needed somewhere to go) and so now, he wants to do one, too! My 2½-year-old likes smoothies just fine ("moothie!") and that's even with chard!

—*Steffanie D.*

I started drinking green smoothies almost three years ago and lost over 30 pounds, regained my health, and felt 10 years younger. My children never need visits to the doctor unless they have been injured. The evidence is so obvious that I cannot ever cease this miracle drink.

—*Julie Greenman*

My husband and I have been enjoying green smoothies 6–7 times a week for the past 9 months. We are hooked! In fact, we went on vacation for a week and missed our Blendtec blender and green smoothie so much, we could hardly wait to get back home to start again. My husband was diagnosed with bladder cancer three years ago, and the doctor consistently was removing new tumor sites every three months.

Once we found GreenSmoothieGirl.com, got our blender, and started making the smoothies, he has consistently been clear of any new tumors. His latest colonoscopy this year was also clear, he has more energy, and feels healthy and strong. We will not go without our healthy green start each day! We can't thank you enough!

—*Nancy K.*

I have hyperthyroid (Graves' Disease) and have been on Propyl-Thyracil (PTU) for the past 15 years. During this time, doctors and specialists have urged me to go on radioactive iodine, and some of them have even ridiculed me for wanting to consider alternative methods.

I knew instinctively that an answer lay for me in something else besides pills. But I was told that they knew of nothing else and that the iodine treatment was pretty standard. (Well, not for me, thank you very much!) I have searched and searched for years. I even went off PTU for three months thinking that I could use positive thinking and visualization to heal myself...but to no avail.

So when I came across green smoothies in June 2008, I knew that it was more like a liquid salad, full of nutrition and basic goodness. Together with beginning a high raw food lifestyle, I was able to decrease my PTU intake every 3 months since then, when having an appointment with my endocrinologist to check out blood work. I had been on three PTUs per day.

After the first three months, I decreased it to two, thinking that there would be some changes to my blood work results. Since there was none, again after three months, I decreased it to one PTU per day. Again, no changes in T4, Free T3, and sTSH results. My last appointment with the endocrinologist was in January 2009. Again, no changes.

She was delighted and suggested that I come off PTU completely. I almost fell off my chair that a doctor would suggest no pills. Of my own choice, and with her approval, I asked if I should consider half a PTU per day until my next appointment. She agreed. To date, I feel fine with no increased palpitation and an abundance of energy. Thank you so much green smoothies and, most of all, thank you to Robyn for her relentless pursuit of research.

—*Hal Walter; Ottawa, Ontario, Canada*

After a year of thinking and searching deeply about going vegetarian, I took the leap in September 2008. What made the transition easy was the discovery of the green smoothie! I first heard of them on Robyn's informative website, GreenSmoothie Girl.com. I was intrigued and investigated the origins of green smoothies and started to find whole blogging communities who were drinking these liquid vegetable treats. I viewed many of the YouTube videos Robyn had posted and saw how simple it was to get my veggies the green smoothie way. I started right away, using my simple kitchen blender. My 11-year-old son and my husband were curious and started drinking them with me almost immediately. We *love* them!

The chronic eczema around the edges of my scalp are clearing up (some are completely gone!), ridges in my fingernails are flattening out and the nails have become hard, chronic tiredness has been replaced with vibrant energy, mild arthritic symptoms in fingers vanished, hypothyroid symptoms growing less (although I'm on a low dose of Armour and have been for years, I still experience many of the hypothyroid symptoms—but they are really improving!), insomnia seems to be vanquished, I've lost 9 pounds so far, and I don't know if this could be related but I no longer sunburn!

But what is truly amazing is I'm growing in streaks of brown hair where it was solid silver before—fabulous!

We are experiencing great health benefits from these marvelous drinks and I think we may be addicted to the vibrancy and high-energy kick we get from them. I'll be getting results from a blood test next week and I can't wait to see the numbers! I've turned several friends and family members into green smoothie drinkers and am actually pursuing a radio show where I will be able to discuss and share my progress with others. Thank you, Robyn, for GreenSmoothieGirl blogs! Your generosity in sharing your info with the world has inspired so many to move toward health!

—*Cher*

I love them, I love green smoothies anyway, and I love your recipes the best. It is so good to have mainly greens and a few fruits instead of the other way around as I was previously doing. I love them and my kids do also. They crave them as I do.

—*Anon.*

My New Year's Resolution was to Go Green. My husband and I (yes, I converted him) both love the green smoothies. They are very satisfying. We no longer crave junk food. We have begun to lose a few pounds. I am turning on my grandchildren and children to them. My husband is Hispanic, diabetic, high cholesterol, and high blood pressure. We are seeing improvements. It has only been a month. We use our Blendtec for breakfast, lunch, and dinner. We make smoothies, salad dressings, and soups and using your *12 Steps to Whole Foods* book each month, we aim to be totally green after one year. Thank you for all your research and recipes.

—*Pat M.*

Green smoothies became a part of my life at the same time that I started eating 100 percent raw. So the effects are probably due to raw food (which green smoothies are) in general. I do know that the effects have been real for me, and I refer everyone I possibly can to GreenSmoothieGirl.com so they can reap the benefits, too.

Many people do not want to go all raw, but they can improve by adding green smoothies, and eating more raw foods. I was able to quit taking oral medications for diabetes after making these changes and have been stable without medications for almost a year now. I am looking forward to even more improvements as I continue on this path. I am so grateful for Robyn and for the contribution she has made to the community in helping people understand this vital information. I am convinced that health and longevity is based on what we put in and on our bodies, and that we are responsible for our own health and vitality. If we are not willing to do what is necessary, Nature will impose the consequences.

—*DJSK*

Green smoothies have helped me stay full longer in the morning. I used to be *so* hungry by lunchtime. My stomach would growl and I would become dizzy. Now I drink a blender full of smoothie in the morning and I am satisfied until it is time to eat my next meal.

—*J. Burns*

My day is not complete without a smoothie! If I go without one, I feel bad physically and mentally. My children love them, too, and want them every day so they can have energy and strong muscles.

—*Jenny L.*

I've been drinking a quart of green smoothies daily for about a year now, with a few exceptions. When I fail to drink them for a few days (too busy, need to go to the store, etc.), I find that the first sip of the next smoothie is so welcome, so delicious, so satisfying.

My children drink them because I put them in front of them. I gave them a pint at first, and my 11-year-old son struggled to get them down. I let him drink half a pint for a while, until he got used to it. Finally, he asked if he still had to drink the small glass (half a pint), or if he could have a full glass now—*yes*! He also enjoys drinking them in front of friends and telling them what's in it. That took a couple of weeks, probably.

Now, they drink a pint, and sometimes whatever else is leftover after I have mine. They like lots of strawberries in theirs, and fresh peaches, when they're in season. I have converted several friends to drinking green smoothies, too. (Them: "What is that you're drinking?" Me: "A green smoothie." Them: "What's in it?" Me: "Want a taste?" or "Would you like the recipe?")

—*Janelle B.*

I purchased my Blendtec Total Blender at Costco during a demo at the store. The demo guy recommended I go online to GreenSmoothieGirl.com for great recipes and support. Since I have been drinking the green smoothie, my bowels are more regular than they have ever been. I was diagnosed with Irritable Bowel Syndrome and now I do not have constipation. It is the most wonderful feeling to be regular! Also, since adding the dark leafy green vegetables, I have been able to avoid colds from grandkids and friends. I can honestly say I am much healthier. I never miss a day and it has been about 4 months. Thank you, Robyn.

—*Barbara A.*

I started doing smoothies twice a day (breakfast and lunch), July 14, 2008. At the time, I had no idea what to expect, as I was just trying this on a whim. After about two weeks, I noticed I lost about 5 pounds. I decided to continue this process, and switching up my dinners to be cooked, mostly vegetarian. Another 2–3 weeks passed by and I lost another 5 pounds. Something was working...I suspect it was the combination of green smoothies and going mostly vegetarian.

Well, along my journey, I started seeing books about raw food and 80-10-10, and just a whole bunch of information. I decided to try doing raw, and for the most part I have been able to maintain about 90–95 percent raw since I started doing this. Every week that passed I noticed I kept losing 2.5 pounds a week, for an eventual total loss so far of about 47 pounds. About 3 months into my journey, I read *80-10-10 Diet* by Douglas Graham, and have implemented a lot of his concepts in my daily routines, so most of my daily intake consists of fruits and vegetables, with very small amounts of nuts and seeds. I noticed that with gourmet raw using high content fat (i.e., nuts and seeds), I would do alright but I truly thrived doing 80-10-10.

As far as exercise goes, even before I started smoothies, twice a week at the gym I was doing a cycle/spin class, and I would occasionally do some light weights at home. I have noticed that in my cycle/spin classes, I have been able to maintain extremely high energy levels and not gas out when on 80-10-10. I also noticed that when doing raw-gourmet (with higher fat), that I would not be as energized. Another thing I should note, my muscle recovery times have improved dramatically with 80-10-10—gone are the days of recovery, instead my muscle recovery occurs in about 15–20 hours, ready to hit up more exercise the next day.

I used to have a sinus headache about once a week. Those are all gone. I sleep much better, and noticed that I can go on my day with less sleep and still have a ton of energy. My daily diet still consists of two smoothies a day (one breakfast and one lunch) and my typical dinner meal varies, but it is typically in line with 80-10-10. It took me about 6 months to lose nearly 50 pounds, but the whole process was pretty easy. It is just a matter of committing your mind, and making great habits and breaking the bad ones.

—*Eddie Yee*

I really enjoy green smoothies, but the biggest surprise to me is that my husband loves them even more than I do. He does not really care for vegetables, so it is totally shocking to me that he waits around in the morning until I make him a smoothie and gives me crazy feedback like "this is too sweet, it needs more kale!" or "this needs more ginger." It is awesome!

—*Kendra A.*

I had a complete CBC analysis done in April 2008—just 2 months before I started the green smoothies and then I had it done again in October 2008, 4 months after starting. Here are some interesting results:

April 2008 – These were all in the high range:

Cholesterol – 267

Cholesterol HDL Ratio – 7.9

LDL Cholesterol – 201

Glucose – 117

Triglycerides – 161

October 2008 – These were all in the normal range:

Cholesterol – 181

Cholesterol HDL ratio – 4.8

LDL Cholesterol – 116

Glucose – 91

Triglycerides – 136

—*Bonnie E.*

I have spent all my adulthood overweight and miserable. My weight went from 135 to 280 during that time. Most of the time I had skewed ideas that I was either too fat (when I weighed 135) and not that fat (when I weighed 280). My perception was always off. But I did know that I just didn't feel good.

I have been on Weight Watchers, the soup diet, hard boiled egg diet, Chinese tea, and every diet that came in magazines. I finally found that Atkins worked for me—three times! Funny that I would go off after several months and the weight would come back on, with its 30-pound friend! I realized that if I kept dieting that way I would completely ruin my health. I was so afraid to start another diet, I decided to never diet again and just accept myself as I was.

I remarried at 210 pounds and within 3 years had put on 70 pounds with careless eating, primarily fast food. Then my DH was diagnosed with cancer (digestive related) and I found GreenSmoothieGirl.com. It was an answer to prayer because this is a *lifestyle*—not a diet. In the last 9 months I have lost 40 pounds, my skin glows, I am nearly off the medications I was taking for high blood pressure, arthritic aches and pains, and mucus. My wrinkles also are going away!

I will *never* diet again because I can eat everything I want and truly enjoy it (even chocolate). I am never hungry because I have God's fast food with me all the time (fruits). I have found that the more raw I eat, the faster I lose weight. I am no longer fanatical about it and believe that my body will end up the weight I am supposed to be, not the way society says it should be. I just wish I had been able to learn this earlier in life.

Sorry about the long message, but I feel that finding Green SmoothieGirl.com and Robyn's blog has saved my life! Thanks,

Robyn, and everyone else!

—*Karen L.*

My husband and I began with the green smoothies with Robyn in February 2008. Within three months my husband lost 60 pounds and I have kept off 20 and am at my normal weight ... what I have averaged since high school. I am 5'4" and 108. I am 41 and have two children under the age of 5. My husband can now sleep through the night (he used to toss and turn). I sleep soundly. I close my eyes and it is morning! My husband no longer needs Prilosec. My children, 2½ and 5, drink green smoothies and they have not been sick in a year. My son goes to a special-needs school and I have noticed that his behavior is much better. He also has an amazing creative streak in the past 6 months. Thank you, Robyn!

—*Tonya Carney*

Both my 18-year-old daughter and 15-year-old son are hooked! My daughter used to pass out with fatigue after school every day for the last 3 years but not now, and she has only 16 ounces for breakfast. My son has 16 ounces for breakfast, and after one week he asked if he could *please* take a quart for school lunch every day! His energy is now what it should be and he no longer craves starchy/white/dead carbohydrates and wants to eat better also. The cracked, dry, sore spots at each side of his mouth (almost looked like small tear or split/cracked creases on both sides) have gone for good.

That old afternoon fatigue and sugar craving and a nap is history and coffee addiction of 10 years is gone, along with the deep face creases caused by it all! Most exciting is lifelong bad breath has disappeared, and who knows what other marvels are happening inside? It's only been 30 days!

—*Susan W.*

I'm always constipated, and I used to drink herbal laxatives to help me, but they give me terrible abdominal cramps and diarrhea. Drinking green smoothie four days a week has helped me a lot. I feel great!

—*Anon.*

Green smoothies have impacted my life in so many ways. I had gained 65 pounds from my first pregnancy on my "organic" processed-food diet. My self-esteem and confidence were crumbling around me. My energy levels ran on low even though I am only in my 20s. I remember when I was introduced to the concept of green smoothies at a health food store. A lady was handing out free samples. I used to work at a smoothie bar and the thought of adding greens to smoothies had never occurred to me.

It was two years ago when I discovered this amazing drink, and I have had one every day since. People started to comment on how "radiant" my skin looked and asked how I was losing weight only 2–3 months after starting green smoothies. Soon, I had to make a printout of recipes and tips to give out to friends and family to make explaining the "green smoothie" easier and not as redundant. Not long after that, I started teaching health classes. There are probably more families at my church making smoothies than those that are not. We have all seen a difference in our health. I do not crave salty and sweet things like I used to. I feel like the chains of my cravings were released with the key of smoothies.

I have lost over 40 pounds and gained soaring levels of energy. I have a better outlook on life. I prefer to go for a walk instead of watching TV with a bag of chips by my side. My passion has grown so much for this simple concept that I am working on a website called www.smoothie-handbook.com. I want others to feel the freedom that I am experiencing.

In February 2009, I had my second son. Thank goodness I can say that I didn't gain 65 pounds this time around—only 16! I lost all of that on delivery day. Even though I didn't gain a lot of weight, my 9-pound newborn was not lacking in that area. By 6 weeks post-partum, I was 6 pounds under my pre-pregnancy weight! I was not starving myself, either. The green smoothies give me so many different nutrients that my body doesn't crave the junk.

I am so glad that there are people like Robyn out there promoting such a wonderful concept. Because of people like her, I am a totally different person. Thank you!

—*DaNae Johnson*

I have been drinking green smoothies daily for a month now. I have seen a huge improvement in my overall outlook on life. I handle stress *so* much better and I feel happier. Another huge improvement for me was the decrease in my cravings for sugary foods. This was a big problem for me. Now even if I eat something sweet, I don't want very much of it. It has been amazing how much better I feel since starting to drink green smoothies!

—*Tammy M.*

My wife and I have noticeably improved skin tone and clearer complexion and have had people notice and make comments. We noted some indigestion during the day as we added both fruit and vegetables to our smoothies that digest differently, but was minor. We also weren't very hungry for 4–5 hours after drinking the green smoothie.

—*Scott*

My husband and I have always tried to eat healthy, but adding green smoothies to our daily routine has made it so much easier. A 20-ounce smoothie for breakfast sets the day for us. Both of us used to have major carb cravings, and my husband also craved a lot of sugar, but when we start the day with a green smoothie, neither of us experience these cravings (unless we allow ourselves to get *really* hungry).

My 2-year-old son loves green smoothies as well. He has never had the junk food that a lot of kids his age are so accustomed to, so I wouldn't call adding smoothies to his diet a "conversion," but I'm still impressed every day when he gulps his down and asks for more.

Thanks, Robyn, for preaching the Gospel of Green. We are converted for life!

—*Mandi L.*

We've been converted to green smoothies for a while now. In fact, I'll have to say that I crave them. Not necessarily the taste (although our concoction is very tasty), but the effects they have on me! I feel so much healthier and my skin tone has definitely improved. People tell me I look so young—who doesn't like to hear that?! My daughter and grandson are hooked now, too. Thanks Robyn!

—*Karen P.*

The symptoms I experienced for years are almost too long to list, everything from diabetes to back pain to asthma to an all-over deep muscle pain and nerve problems (tingling, burning, numbness, etc.). Most symptoms have disappeared altogether or been significantly reduced. I had used green smoothies off and on for a couple of years, but went heavy on them plus switched to an all-raw diet at the end of July last year.

—*Anon.*

I am using green smoothies and raw foods to kick a 15-year drinking habit and it's working! Green smoothies and organic, raw foods are changing my body at the cellular level and I definitely feel it! And what's wonderful is that, unlike some pills, I can feel the results immediately. The same day!

My emotional health has greatly improved. I am positive, hopeful, and my self-esteem is increasing. Sometimes two green smoothies are all I need all day long, not even hungry at night! It's fun to try different recipes, and I have two bottles I use just for my green drinks and smoothies. I feel really good knowing that I'm cleansing and healing my body with green smoothies. I'm even planning to make green smoothies when I travel, as long as I'm able to use a blender wherever I go!

The people I have tried to convert are just really skeptical. I keep telling them that they are delicious and that if you use a couple bananas, a mango, and handful or two of spinach that it tastes sweet and fruity, no "green" taste at all! But personally, I really enjoy savory smoothies just as much as a fruit smoothie! I'm so excited about your new book, Robyn! Great job!

—*Jennie W*

I had pain in both knees for about 20 years and after drinking the green smoothie for 30 days, I can now walk down a hill or downstairs without as much pain. Also the pain that I had from fibromyalgia is disappearing.

—*Jackie H.*

I began drinking a quart of green smoothie daily when I was about eight months pregnant. I felt so healthy for the remainder of the pregnancy, regained my strength quickly after a long labor, and shed my pregnancy weight in less than six weeks. Now, more than a year later, I have lost an additional 30 pounds and feel great. I firmly believe that anyone who is seriously trying to lose weight in a healthy way should be drinking green smoothies. Green smoothies are now a permanent fixture in my family's diet. We drink them for breakfast, for snacks, and with our occasional breakfast-for-dinner meals. My older child enjoys sharing them with playmates, and we've even brought a full pitcher of smoothie to a potluck with a breakfast theme. I've yet to meet a person who tries a green smoothie and doesn't enjoy it.

—*Tina H.*

I love everything about green smoothies. They have made a great improvement in my life. I share them with anyone interested in tasting one and most everyone loves them as much as I do! People who are not open-minded enough to try a small taste, well, they do not know what a grand, life-changing experience they are missing. I was so excited when my 21-year-old daughter told me about green smoothies. I could not wait to try one. What an awesome gift to share with anyone that you love!!!

—*Bonnie K.*

I was diagnosed with breast cancer in 1999. I had a surgery to remove the lump but refused chemo and radiation. I saw a naturopathic doctor and through microwater, stabilizing my pH, and diet, was able to get rid of it. In the spring of 2008 I knew from the symptoms the cancer was back.

I checked my pH, which was so acidic it wouldn't even read on the paper. I went to see my doctor and he confirmed the readings. I knew the key to getting rid of cancer was a balanced pH. I have a microwater machine, but I knew the fastest way to balance pH is through greens, but it was impossible to eat the amount that I needed.

I've been drinking blended greens faithfully since August 2008 along with the raw food, no dairy, no meat. I was rechecked for cancer in January and there are no signs at all. I feel great, haven't been sick. I've lost weight and am back down to my high school weight and size. I have energy, etc....I could go on and on. My kids can't believe I'm running around chasing the grandkids like a teenager. The green drink is the best breakfast a person could have.

Because of the positive change in me, about 10 other people have started drinking green smoothies. Ladies at Curves, my husband, my daughter, my husbands' parents, my parents, and my friends. And when I go to Sunflower Market, I meet a lot of people, mostly older people buying kale for their green drink. I smile and think, wow, that's great!

—*Terri Barnett, Payson, Utah*

When I slow down on drinking green smoothies, it seems my joints start getting stiff and I get tired again. Also I stop being regular and go back to bowel movements once every three days!

—*Anon.*

My 2 youngest drink green smoothies almost every morning for breakfast. They even share some of it at school and some of the kids have asked for the recipe. Out of my eight children they have the nicest skin even though they do eat some junk food out of the home. The others get acne really bad. This is amazing! I just noticed when the youngest was away with his friends for a few days his face started breaking out again. I don't think this is a coincidence. He asked for green smoothies when he got back.

—*Althea*

We drink green smoothies daily as a family. Even my 8-year-old likes them and he is a soccer player convinced it helps with his game skills. Thank you!

—*Laura W.*

Love my green smoothies. When I drink them I am not as hungry and feel when I do eat I need to eat nutritionally dense foods, not fake foods. I have nice skin, hair, nails and a good deal of energy.

—*Wendy K.*

I started making green smoothies a year ago. My husband had been diagnosed with hemochromatosis several years earlier. He had gotten that under control but because the disease had gone undiagnosed for years, he had organ damage, including heart, liver, and kidney. He had no energy. So he started every day with a 2-liter bottle of Mountain Dew. My mission was to get him off the Mountain Dew and replace it with something that was better for him and gave him the energy he needed.

After some research and finding GreenSmoothieGirl.com, I purchased a high-speed blender. I started making green smoothies every day. I persuaded my husband to get off the caffeine and sugar and give this a try. He has done remarkably well. I went into this hoping, but knowing how difficult it is to break such an entrenched habit of caffeine. I had my doubts.

I am happy to report after one year, he has not gone back to Mountain Dew and he feels more energetic than he has in the last several years. I also have felt the benefits of green smoothies. Although starting this in generally good health, I feel better, more energetic and have better digestion than I have felt in years. A year ago I also stopped cooking meat for dinner every night. Although we have not gone to a 100 percent vegan diet, we have cut out 75 percent of the meat we used to eat. I am trying to cook healthier and have used Robyn's recipes to do that. All that I have tried have been very good. I would recommend this simple lifestyle change to everyone.

—*Karen R.*

In spring 2006, I gained 30 pounds in 6 weeks when I started taking a particular birth control pill. Of course I went off of it, but it seemed to push me into some major perimenopause symptoms including depression, exhaustion, and continued weight gain. I went to several doctors who tried various hormone treatments, thyroid treatment, the candida diet and treatment—all of which seemed to make me worse!

So in the spring 2007, I decided to take matters into my own hands. I stopped all medications and diets and began to treat myself with food and exercise. I committed myself to try it for a year and just see what happened. I felt desperate, so I decided to just eat mostly raw fruits and vegetables, believing that they were the cleansing and building tools my body needed. I made up the green smoothie on my own and started drinking it all day and supplementing it with veggies and at night a potato and sometimes a little meat and cooked veggie. For eight months there was no change in my weight, but I did start feeling much better and at least I stopped gaining weight!

My hot flashes almost completely stopped, and in January 2008, I finally lost 15 pounds all at once. One day one of my clients told me about greensmoothiegirl.com when she saw me with a huge mug of green stuff. I went home that night and looked it up and have been a huge fan ever since! I was so glad to have support and new ideas and information.

I don't think I have completely solved my health problems, because I'm sure my thyroid is still very sluggish, and I still can't get that last 15 pounds off, but I feel so much better. Now I am committed to eat this way the rest of my life just for the health of it!

I love green smoothies and having an easy way to get so many veggies in that I would never eat otherwise. You could say I am an addict! I love them mostly because of the way I begin to feel (sluggish and run-down) when I have to go without them for very many days. I have been doing them for a year and a half and it feels like my body is slowly but surely repairing from many years of not having enough live enzymes. My hot flashes are almost nonexistent when I drink my greens.

The protein in the leafy greens keeps me from being hungry till afternoon. Anyone who knows me knows that I am a green smoothie freak. Many have told me that I inspire them to want to eat more healthfully. I have taught many people how to make them, and my mom and husband are as committed to having them as I am. My husband ran the Boston Marathon last year (at 52 years old) without the benefit of green smoothies. Since October he has had them 4 or 5 days a week, and we are anxious to see if he improves his performance this year. We will let you know!

—*Debbie W.*

P.S. When I give my grandchildren tastes of my green smoothies, they love it! Now I just need to get their parents committed.

I feel a major decrease in cravings for sweets. I have lost some weight, nothing major, but that is not my primary goal. I am a runner and have noticed a difference in my endurance and performance. I feel healthier and cleaner. I am hooked for life and my days aren't the same when I don't get my normal 32 ounces! I got my mom and my toddler hooked. My son calls them "mooshies" and begs for them all throughout the day. He would keep one in his hand all day long if I'd let him. I'm excited to continue to drink green smoothies and improve my life as well as my family's.

—*Meghan Meredith*

I work for a lady who began eating raw. As I watched her transform, I became very interested in what she was doing and remembered how good I used to feel when I was younger and ate and drank more raw food. I asked her a lot of questions and began to follow a healthier raw eating and drinking plan, beginning with a green smoothie every morning.

I have two teenage daughters who joined in with me on this path of health. One of them has become very disciplined with her eating habits and loves this way of enjoying our food. She has lost all of her baby fat and her skin has cleared up. She is an athlete and very involved in sports. She said that now that she drinks green she can make it through the class day without falling asleep!

We all feel better and I have stopped taking all allergy meds and asthma inhalers.

—*Heidi Underwood*

I'm 17 and a raw vegan and green smoothies have changed my life! I always felt tired and cranky and always a little hungry but as soon as I added green smoothies, I felt awesome! They give me everything I need. I love my green smoothies!

—*Brendon Clarke-Pepper*

Green smoothies have changed my life. Not only have I converted my family members, but also the people I work with. My 15-month-old son loves the green smoothies and always asks for more. I feel better, look better, and love that I was able to spread the word about green smoothie goodness!

—*Jamie Stavinaha*

My name is Kathy Wells and I love green smoothies. My youngest daughter is 6 and she also loves them now. My oldest is working on them. But I have been able to convert her into eating healthy fruits and veggies. So her smoothies have less green in them but they are getting better.

—*Kathy W.*

You are a fountain of information for the newbie.

As you mention on one of your blog posts, I had slowly been feeling uncomfortable with what I eat, as if I'm not really feeding my body, just putting empty calories into it. Obvious malnutrition. As soon as I discovered green smoothies, I have had a newfound sense of clarity, the ever-present fog has lifted from my head, and I have changed the way I eat without even being aware of it.

All cravings for junk—chocolate, refined carbs, etc.—have vanished. Not easy here in New York, where you are bombarded with all and everything all the time. I have never eaten fast food, and not really a red meat eater, but am in the habit of grabbing convenient processed foods—completely full of chemicals and preservatives. No wonder after doing 1 day of green smoothies, I had detox headaches all day. Ha!

I recently bought recipes from your site, but just want to say thanks for such informed and detailed information for those of us out there getting started. You are on the top of my bookmark list.

—*Alexia*

I have had such amazing results from green smoothies, that I have converted my boyfriend Steve and he has converted his mom and brother (he's still working on his dad). We feel more energized, we have lost weight—almost 20 pounds between us, no cravings for sweets (never saw that coming), greatly reduced appetite, and much clearer skin. It has really inspired us to be more proactive in working toward optimal health.

We now research every restaurant before we go out, due to the fattiness in the food/unhealthy ingredients. We are severely limited on where we will eat now outside the house. We are pretty limited to sushi places, as the food is prepared fresh and the sushi is raw and they are our favorite, anyway!

We are eating way more fruits and veggies than normal, and we have actually developed cravings for greens! We are also barely eating meat outside of fish, and have even gone organic! I want to thank you for your insight and all your information on this site.

When I first read about and got into smoothies around November 2008, it was your YouTube videos I watched to learn about this new way of life. It was your site that gave me my first green smoothie recipes, and helped me on my path to health. I also bought the Blendtec, which is my prized possession! I have even made "ice cream" in it. It's amazing. Well worth the time it took to save up the money for it! I use it at least 2 times a day. Thank you again for everything and good luck with the new book. I'll be anxiously awaiting it!

—*Jenny; Staten Island, New York*

Index

Other Books from Ulysses Press

The Green Smoothie Bible: 300 Delicious Recipes
Kristine Miles, $14.95

More than 300 inviting recipes in *The Green Smoothie Bible* show how to combine leafy green vegetables and delicious, antioxidant-rich fruits into the most nutritious drinks imaginable—leaving you healthy and feeling amazing inside and out.

Green Smoothie Cleanse: Detox, Lose Weight and Maximize Good Health with the World's Most Powerful Superfoods
Lisa Sussman, $14.95

Unleash the power of leafy greens for a one-of-a-kind cleanse that doesn't leave you starved or deprived. The easy-to-follow program in this book packs key vitamins, minerals and antioxidants into tasty and healing smoothies.

Green Smoothies for Every Season: A Year of Farmers Market–Fresh Super Drinks
Kristine Miles, $16.95

Capable of transforming your health in remarkable ways, leafy greens and fresh fruits are vital for living well and feeling great. *Green Smoothies for Every Season* provides the most effective way to harness the power of these antioxidant-rich superfoods with organic, fresh smoothies you make at home.

To order these books call 800-377-2542 or 510-601-8301, fax 510-601-8307, e-mail ulysses@ulyssespress.com, or write to Ulysses Press, P.O. Box 3440, Berkeley, CA 94703. All retail orders are shipped free of charge. California residents must include sales tax. Allow two to three weeks for delivery.

FREE OFFER FOR
The Green Smoothies Diet readers only:

Please get my 20-page GreenSmoothieGirl *12 Nutrition Myths Special Report* about things you have likely believed your whole life that are hurting your health. Learn how to spot false doctrine in the world of nutrition. With this simple knowledge, you can quickly learn more and make better food choices than 99 percent of your peers in the Western world. These myths are well-documented in scientific literature, but you won't read about them in the mainstream media! Go here to get this important special report, free:

http://www.12NutritionMyths.com

Testimonials for Robyn's *12 Nutrition Myths*:

My husband and I have been reading your *12 Myths* with astonishment, and researching to learn that you're right about all of it! We believed every single one of these myths for over 50 years! As we incorporate this new information, our weight is decreasing and our health and energy is improving. Please keep sharing this information—we wish we had it sooner but are so grateful!
—Evelyn M.; Texas

I've been checking out all your *12 Myths*, many of which my doctor told me are true. Now I'm mad because YOU'RE RIGHT, and I've been told wrong by people I trusted. I found lots of sources for this information online and in books. I'm telling everyone I know about this report. It's like the lightbulb just went on in my brain. Now I'm rethinking everything I put in my grocery cart.
—James M.; California

About the Author

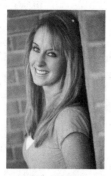

Robyn Openshaw is a nutrition enthusiast and educator whose previous work includes *12 Steps to Whole Foods*. She has a following on GreenSmoothieGirl.com, YouTube, and Facebook, and her biggest passion is helping young moms ("They change the world!") feed their families a whole-food, plant-based, mostly raw diet. She is part-time faculty at Brigham Young University and a single mom to four competitive athletes, two boys and two girls. She loves to play competitive tennis, snow ski, run outside, grow organic vegetables, cook (i.e., "arrange the elements"), and read everything in sight. She lives in Lindon, Utah.